DATE DUE

FAMILIES WITH HANDICAPPED MEMBERS

James C. Hansen, Editor
Evan Imber Coppersmith, Volume Editor

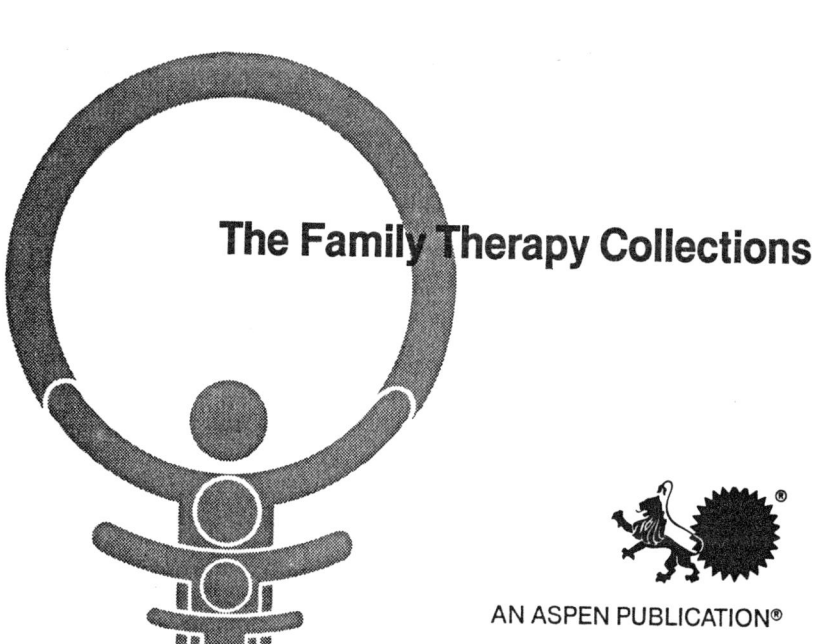

The Family Therapy Collections

AN ASPEN PUBLICATION®

Aspen Systems Corporation
Rockville, Maryland
Royal Tunbridge Wells
1984

Library of Congress Cataloging in Publication Data
Main entry under title:

Families with handicapped members.

(The Family therapy collections, ISSN: 0735-9152; 11)
Includes bibliographies.
1. Handicapped — Mental health services — Addresses, essays, lectures.
2. Handicapped children — Mental health services — Addresses, essays, lectures. 3. Handicapped — Home care — Addresses, essays, lectures.
4. Handicapped — children — Home care — Addresses, essays, lectures.
5. Handicapped — Family relationships — Addresses, essays, lectures.
6. Handicapped children — Family relationships — Addresses, essays, lectures. 7. Family therapy — Addresses, essays, lectures. I. Hansen, James C. II. Coppersmith, Evan Imber. III. Series.
RC451.4.H35F36   1984   362.8'286   84-12315
ISBN: 0-89443-612-0

Publisher: John R. Marozsan
Associate Publisher: Jack W. Knowles, Jr.
Editorial Director: Margaret Quinlin
Executive Managing Editor: Margot G. Raphael
Managing Editor: M. Eileen Higgins
Editorial Services: Ruth McKendry
Printing and Manufacturing: Debbie Collins

The Family Therapy Collections series is indexed in *Psychological Abstracts* and the PsycINFO database.

Copyright © 1984 by Aspen Systems Corporation

All rights reserved. This book, or parts thereof, may not be reproduced in any form or by any means, electronic or mechanical, including photocopy, recording, or any information storage and retrieval system now known or to be invented, without written permission from the publisher, except in the case of brief quotations embodied in critical articles or reviews. For information, address Aspen Systems Corporation, 1600 Research Boulevard, Rockville, Maryland 20850.

Library of Congress Catalog Card Number: 84-12315
ISBN: 0-89443-612-0
ISSN: 0735-9152

Printed in the United States of America

Table of Contents

Board of Editors vii

Contributors ix

Preface xi

Introduction xiii

1. **Families with Infants and Young Children Who Have Special Needs** 1
   Janine Roberts

   Review of Literature 2
   Family Reaction 4
   Guidelines for Therapists 7
   Developmental Life Cycle Issues 7
   Larger Systems 10
   Guidelines for Therapists 12
   Family Adaptation 13
   Guidelines for Therapists 15
   Conclusion 15

2. Working with Families of School-Aged Handicapped Children 18
Lee Combrinck-Graham and L. Wayne Higley

Family Life Cycle 19
Family Patterns 21
Role of Family Therapy 22
Conclusion 28

3. From Home to College, From College to Home: An Interactional Approach to Treating the Symptomatic Disabled College Student 30
Richard A. Whiting, Linda L. Terry, and Helyn Strom-Henriksen

Traditional Perspective 31
An Interactional Approach 32
Characteristics of Families with a Symptomatic
    Disabled Member 35
Clinical Considerations 38
Conclusion 41

4. Bearing the Burden Alone? Helping Divorced Mothers of Children with Developmental Disabilities 44
Lynn Wikler, Jane Haack, and James Intagliata

Stresses of Divorced Mothers of Children with
    Developmental Disabilities 46
Family Interventions 52

5. Relationships of the Handicapped: Issues of Sexuality and Marriage 63
Gary L. Sanders

Definition of Handicap 64
The Impact of Disability 64
Basic Assumptions 65
Clinical Evaluation 66
Intervention: Plissit 68
Conclusion 73

6. **The Elderly and Their Families:**
   An Interactional View 75
   Wendy L. Watson and Lorraine M. Wright

   Physiological Problems of Aging 76
   Psychological Problems of Aging 78
   Problems of Aging and the Family 78
   Interactional Aspects of Aging 80

7. **Frames and Reframing** 88
   Steve de Shazer and Eve Lipchik

   Frames and Reframing 89
   Case Example 90
   Discussion 96
   Conclusion 96

8. **Mobilization: A Natural Resource of the Family** 98
   Sam Scott

   Therapist's Role 99
   Family #1 100
   Family #2 105
   Conclusion 109

9. **A Social Action Perspective: The Disabled and Their**
   Families in Context 111
   Laurie MacKinnon and Nancy Marlett

   Paradigms of Social Problems 112
   The Changing Social Climate 115
   Implications of a Social Action Perspective 119
   Conclusion 125

10. **Social Network Interventions for Families That**
    Have a Handicapped Child 127
    Michael Berger

    Interventions to Preserve Network Integrity 129
    Family Problem Solving 132
    Network Meetings as a Context for Enactments 134
    Engaging Network Members in Treatment 135
    Conclusion 136

11. **Retarded Adults, Their Families, and Larger Systems: A New Role for the Family Therapist** **138**
    Stephen Bloomfield, Scott Nielsen, and Lauren Kaplan

    The Problem 140
    Recommendations 146
    Conclusion 149

12. **A Special "Family" with Handicapped Members: One Family Therapist's Learnings from the L'Arche Community** **150**
    Evan Imber Coppersmith

    L'Arche: A Brief Historical Overview 151
    L'Arche, Calgary: A Systemic Analysis 152
    Implications for the Family Therapist 158

Board of Editors

Editor
JAMES C. HANSEN
State University of New York at Buffalo
Buffalo, New York

JAMES F. ALEXANDER
University of Utah
Salt Lake City, Utah

CAROLYN L. ATTNEAVE
University of Washington
Seattle, Washington

JOHN ELDERKIN BELL
Stanford University
Palo Alto, California

HOLLIS A. EDWARDS
Toronto East General Hospital
Toronto Family Therapy Institute
Toronto, Ontario, Canada

NATHAN B. EPSTEIN
Brown University
Butler Hospital
Providence, Rhode Island

ALAN S. GURMAN
University of Wisconsin
Medical School
Madison, Wisconsin

JOHN HOWELLS
Institute of Family Psychiatry
Ipswich, England

FLORENCE W. KASLOW
Kaslow Associates, P.A.
West Palm Beach, Florida

DAVID P. KNISKERN
University of Cincinnati
College of Medicine
Central Psychiatric Clinic
Cincinnati, Ohio

LUCIANO L'ABATE
Georgia State Univeristy
Atlanta, Georgia

KITTY LAPERRIERE
Ackerman Institute for Family
Therapy
Columbia University School of
Medicine
New York, New York

ARTHUR MANDELBAUM
The Menninger Foundation
Topeka, Kansas

AUGUSTUS Y. NAPIER
The Family Workshop
Atlanta, Georgia

Board of Editors
(continued)

DAVID H. OLSON
University of Minnesota
St. Paul, Minnesota

VIRGINIA M. SATIR
ANTERRA, Inc.
Menlo Park, California

RODNEY J. SHAPIRO
Veterans Administration Medical Center
San Francisco, California

JUDITH S. WALLERSTEIN
Center for the Family in Transition
Corte Madera, California

CARL A. WHITAKER
University of Wisconsin-Madison
Madison, Wisconsin

ROBERT HENLEY WOODY
University of Nebraska at Omaha
Omaha, Nebraska

Contributors

EVAN IMBER COPPERSMITH, PH.D.
University of Calgary
Calgary, Alberta, Canada

MICHAEL BERGER, PH.D.
Georgia State University
Atlanta, Georgia

STEPHEN BLOOMFIELD, ED.D.
Northamptom Area Mental Health
Services, Inc.
Northamptom, Massachusetts

LEE COMBRINCK-GRAHAM, M.D.
Hahnemann University
Philadelphia, Pennsylvania

STEVE DE SHAZER
Brief Family Therapy Center
Wisconsin Institute on Family Studies
Milwaukee, Wisconsin

JANE HAACK
Madison, Wisconsin

L. WAYNE HIGLEY, PH.D.
Philadelphia Association for Retarded
Citizens
Philadelphia, Pennsylvania

JAMES INTAGLIATA, PH.D.
University of Missouri
Kansas City, Missouri

LAUREN KAPLAN, ED.D.
Hampshire Area Commission on Alcohol
Abuse
Northampton, Massachusetts

EVE LIPCHIK
Brief Family Therapy Center
Wisconsin Institute on Family Studies
Milwaukee, Wisconsin

NANCY MARLETT
University of Calgary
Calgary, Alberta, Canada

LAURIE MACKINNON, M.S.W.
University of Calgary
Calgary, Alberta, Canada

SCOTT NIELSEN, M.ED.
Crossroads Community Growth
Center
Holyoke, Massachusetts

JANINE ROBERTS, ED.D.
University of Massachusetts
Amherst, Massachusetts

GARY SANDERS, M.D.
University of Calgary
Calgary, Alberta, Canada

Contributors
(continued)

SAM SCOTT
Philadelphia Child Guidance Clinic
Philadelphia, Pennsylvania

HELYN STROM-HENRIKSON
Crawford Rehabilitation Services
Bedford, New Hampshire

LINDA TERRY, M.ED.
Springfield College
Springfield, Massachusetts

WENDY WATSON, R.N., PH.D.
University of Calgary
Calgary, Alberta, Canada

RICHARD WHITING, ED.E.
Springfield College
Springfield, Massachusetts

LYNN WIKLER, PH.D.
University of Wisconsin
Madison, Wisconsin

LORRAINE WRIGHT, R.N., PH.D.
University of Calgary
Calgary, Alberta, Canada

Preface

The Family Therapy Collections is a quarterly publication in which topics of current and specific interest to family therapists are reviewed. Each volume serves as a source of information for the practicing therapist by translating theory and research on a single topic in family therapy into practical applications. Authored by practicing professionals, the articles in this volume provide in-depth coverage of families with a handicapped member.

There has been a need for additional information to help therapists understand and work with families that have a handicapped member. This volume does not cover all types of handicaps, but provides concepts of what a handicap is and what it may mean to different families at various stages. There are examples of the impact of a handicapping condition on the individual and the family system. It is apparent that the family's dynamics and behavior are significantly affected by the presence of a handicapped member. A therapist should be knowledgeable about the handicapping condition, the family dynamics, and family-community agency interactions that help or hinder the adjusting process. A significant aspect of this volume is the discussion of the family's involvement with larger systems. In addition to conceptual material, the volume is practical in nature. The articles contain case presentations, descriptions of techniques, and suggestions for the therapist. This is truly a ground-breaking volume in the field.

Evan Imber Coppersmith, Ph.D. is the volume editor. She is Associate Professor and the Coordinator of Training of the Family Therapy Program in the Department of Psychiatry at the University of Calgary, Alberta, Canada. Dr. Coppersmith has made important contributions to the field of family therapy through her work in training programs, consultations with organizations and institutions, and major publications. She has developed a meaningful organization for this volume and selected knowledgeable people to write specific articles. The combination yields a volume with a wealth of information for practitioners.

James C. Hansen
Editor

Introduction

Families with one or more members who are considered "handicapped" face both the ordinary issues that every family faces and those that are idiosyncratic to the particular handicapping condition and its effects on the individual, family interaction, and relationships between the family and the outside world. Family therapists who work with these families require skills in family therapy and knowledge of this population's particular needs. As becomes clear in this volume, the family therapist's work may seem quite different from the therapy usually provided and may require a special inventiveness. A natural respect for family resources, a refusal to focus on so-called deficits or to be lured by labels, and a keen knowledge of complex systemic phenomena are all required when working with families with a handicapped member.

The present volume addresses developmental issues, working with strengths, and the family's involvement with larger systems. The first articles deal with the various stages of the family life cycle of families that have handicapped members. These articles address the salient issues faced by families with handicapped members, and then offer effective examples for working in family therapy. The first article, by Janine Roberts, highlights ways to work with families following the birth of a handicapped infant. This is followed by Lee Combrinck-Graham and Wayne Higley's article focusing on the special issues that families face as their children enter school, such as negotiating with school personnel and adapting to differences that become more apparent as a child interacts with peers. The third article, by Richard Whiting, Linda Terry, and Helyn Strom-Henrikson, speaks to the difficult developmental phase of leaving home and reports on a unique college counseling center's approach to engaging the whole family in a therapy that addresses the changes required by all family members at this stage of life.

Lynn Wikler, Jane Haack, and James Intagliata bring together the particular stresses on single-parent families with handicapped children and describe creative ways to work with such families. The effects of a handicap in an adult on the marital subsystem is dealt with by Gary Sanders. Sanders describes special issues faced by couples when one member is handicapped and offers a treatment model tailored to fit the level of complexity of the problem. Wendy Watson and Lorraine Wright address handicaps in the aging population and their effect on the entire family constellation.

The two articles that focus on family strengths include "Frames and Reframing," by Steve de Shazer and Eve Lipchik, who take a case-centered approach to breaking a "vicious cycle" by creative reframing. In the second article, "Mobilization: A Natural Resource of the Family," Sam Scott addresses the particular ways that a family therapist can discover family resources and channel these for the family coping with a handicapped member.

The final articles deal with families in their wider context, including extended family, helping systems, and cultural attitudes. The articles challenge the family therapist to conceptualize broadly and to intervene at the appropriate systemic level.

Laurie MacKinnon and Nancy Marlett's provocative article calls into question many of our assumptions about family therapy as the correct solution to the problems of families with handicapped members. Michael Berger's article suggests pragmatic approaches that the family therapist can use to intervene between the family and larger systems, including extended family and helping systems. In "Retarded Adults, Their Families, and Larger Systems: A New Role for the Family Therapist," Stephen Bloomfield, Scott Nielson, and Lauren Kaplan reframe the role of a family therapist, describing the therapist as a systemic consultant to the multiple systems involved in the lives of retarded adults. Their work is easily transposed to other age groups and other handicapping conditions that require the interaction of the family and other systems.

The volume concludes with my own piece, "A Special 'Family' with Handicapped Members: One Family Therapist's Learnings from the L'Arche Community," which describes a unique and effective larger system for the handicapped and suggests ways that we, as family therapists, can learn from other systems.

Finally, editing this volume has had special meaning to me, as I am the parent of a child who has developmental disabilities. Jenni is a teen-ager now, and we have lived through many of the events addressed by the authors here. I have been witness to Jenni's struggles and her discovery of differences between herself and others. I have experienced my own turmoil as a parent, always questioning what to accept and what not to accept. I have battled larger systems on her behalf, sometimes successfully, sometimes unsuccessfully. Most important, I have learned from her. Jenni has taught me about courage in the face of great odds, about dignity, about friendship, about focusing on strengths rather than deficits, and about the importance of *being,* as opposed to the importance of doing. Presently, Jenni is a volunteer in a program assisting younger physically and mentally handicapped children. This volume is dedicated to Jennifer Faith Coppersmith.

Evan Imber Coppersmith
Volume Editor

1. Families with Infants and Young Children Who Have Special Needs

Janine Roberts

2 FAMILIES WITH HANDICAPPED MEMBERS

Shortly after birth, the third child born to the family was found to have Down's syndrome. An early childhood service team was immediately called, and a social worker began to work with the family. The parents, shocked and afraid, were trying to sort out the implications of the baby's handicap for their whole family; they asked that the baby go to foster care for an unspecified amount of time. Ten days later, the baby moved home, primarily at the mother's insistence. At this point, they requested therapy, as the mother particularly wanted a place where she could express the range of her feelings and the stresses she was experiencing but was afraid to share with her husband for fear of scaring him more.

A MAJOR PHYSICAL, MENTAL, OR LEARNING HANDICAP AFFECTS 2 OF every 100 babies born in the United States. In addition, the latest figures compiled by the National Center for Health Statistics show that the number of children suffering from chronic illness has doubled, from 1.7% in 1958 to 3.8% in 1981 (Newsweek, August 1, 1983, p. 47). Thus, every year approximately 70,000 families have new babies who have a handicap, and thousands of other families have young children who develop a chronic illness. Yet, this increase in the number of children with special needs is occurring in a "modernized" society in which structural and functional changes in the family often make it more difficult to care for such children (Zisserman, 1981).

Family therapy with families that have an infant or a young child with special needs can be intricate for several reasons. First, there is often uncertainty about the exact nature of the handicap and its implications for the child's future development. Second, families are often involved with a range of social services, and family therapists must carefully define their role with both the families and the agencies. Third, during the initial assessment of the handicap, the time frame seems both compacted and protracted. Parents need to learn to cope day by day with the extra demands of their young child, yet the larger, unknown time frame often intrudes on their thoughts. Families are asking themselves, "What will the future of this family be *now*?"

REVIEW OF LITERATURE

Two distinct kinds of literature on families that have young children with a handicap can be useful to the family therapist: self-report by family members and writings by "professionals." Personal accounts, although biased in that they deal with families that not only have learned to manage the increased familial work and stress associated with raising a child who has special needs, but also have found time to write about it, depict the family perspective and context. Helen Featherstone's book, *A Difference in the Family* (1980) provides both a good overview of these stories, while drawing upon her own family experiences with a severely disabled son from birth to age seven.

Self-report has the benefit of capturing information on one family over time; in contrast, professional literature has the benefit of capturing data on a number of families. Most of the assumptions made in the professional literature are based on case studies or clinical observations of children with specific handicaps and their families, however. As Murphy (1982) noted in her extensive review of the literature "only sixteen of the more than fifty articles reviewed were controlled analytical studies" (p. 73). In most of these research studies, populations with a handicap were compared only with each other; in few studies were families that had children with a handicap compared with a control group that had no children with a handicap (Murphy, 1982). Furthermore, the bulk of the controlled studies involved the parents of moderately to profoundly retarded children.

Little information has been gathered on these families from an interactional perspective. Data have been collected about family dynamics and community relationships only from interviews with the mother (Hewett, 1970; Sultz, Schlesinger, Mosher, & Feldman, 1972; Tropauer, Franz, & Delgard, 1970), from simultaneous but separate interviews with both parents (Farber, 1960), and from questionnaires (Turk, 1964; Weber & Parker, 1981; Wikler, Wasow, & Hatfield, 1981). Significantly fewer fathers than mothers answer questionnaires, however (Gayton, Friedman, Tavormina, & Tucker, 1977; Holroyd, 1974; Holroyd, Brown, Wikler, & Simmons, 1975; McAllister, Butler, & Lei, 1973). Finally, no distinctions have been made in the literature regarding interactive variables, such as congenital versus traumatic etiology of the handicap, age of the child at onset, family size, and income.

A disturbing bias found in some of the professional writing is the emphasis on family dysfunction. This is often highlighted by the language used, e.g., calling the family handicapped (Fotheringham & Cereal, 1974; Sheridan, 1965), describing neuroses and psychotic breaks of parents as common in families that have a child with a handicap (Howell, 1973), discussing the curtailment of parenthood's narcissistic aspects (Murphy, 1982), or labeling family sadness as chronic sorrow (Olshansky, 1962). Two books that are a refreshing change from this stance are Roskies' (1972) work on mothering thalidomide children and Barsch's (1968) interviews with parents of special needs children in Milwaukee.

FAMILY REACTION

Family reaction to a handicap is affected by a number of variables: the nature of the disability and the time of its onset, the family belief system, the affective responses of members, the interface of the family with extended family and other larger systems, and the structure of the family both before and after the onset of the handicap.

Nature and Time of Onset

The severity and visibility of the condition, the remedial prospects, the necessary day-to-day changes in life style, and the time frame of discovery all influence family reaction. For instance, when a handicap is identified at birth, the family may have to deal with a number of diagnostic procedures and interventions shortly after birth, which makes bonding more difficult. The child is clearly defined as different and may be moving in and out of the home for medical care.

A degenerative disease, such as muscular dystrophy, or a disease for which there is no known cure, such as neurofibromatosis, can confront the family with other issues. The family may attain a certain equilibrium and ability to cope with the handicap, only to have the child's condition change. It may be necessary for the family to face the loss of particular capabilities or the death of the child. As one family described their struggle in working with their 4-year-old son who had muscular dystrophy, "Instead of working toward a goal of him improving and getting better, we both know that he is getting worse and there is nothing we can do to prevent it."

When the handicap results from traumatic injury, family members confront a different problem. They must rapidly change their interactions with the child, whom they had previously viewed as "normal." Family members may struggle more directly with the issues of guilt and responsibility (as all parents do at various points), wondering what they might have done differently to protect the child and avoid the injury. Handicaps that have a genetic link may also evoke strong feelings of guilt and responsibility. Family members may protect or blame the parent who may have been the carrier, and issues about further childbearing can become central.

Ambiguity, whether it is around diagnosis, treatment, or prognosis for the handicap, makes the family reaction process more complex. A handicap such as deafness, which may have a clear, treatable course, at least offers the family a focus on which to base actions and expectations. In contrast, a diagnosis of mild retardation offers few clear parameters, so it is difficult to define exactly what is wrong with the child and what may help the child.

Family Belief System

The way in which the family and the outside world frame and understand the reason for the child's handicap and their view of the child's potential also affect the family reaction. The family may view the child with special needs as a gift, feel that they are being punished, or see their experiences as a way to help other families. As the therapist seeks to understand the family belief system, data can be gathered through a series of open-ended questions:

- How do you see the possibilities of the child at this time?
- Where do you see the child 5 years from now?
- What have you told others about the child's problem?
- Who has been most helpful outside of your family? Least helpful?

Knowledge of the family's spiritual and religious context, as well as the ethnic and cultural context (Falicov, 1983; McGoldrick, Pearce, & Giordano, 1982), further helps the therapist to understand what meaning the family gives to the difficulties of the child.

The world view of family members can be an important energizer for the work they do with the child. One family whose child was developmentally delayed framed the problems of the child in this way: "She is delayed 3 months, so therefore if we consider her 9 months old instead of 12, she is normal." This frame served to keep these parents involved and hopeful. The therapist, rather than naming this denial, accepted their view as one that helped them to do all they could for the child.

Affective Responses

A number of theorists have examined the chronological stages of individuals' or families' affective responses to a handicap. Stage theories (Baum, 1962; Klaus & Kennell, 1976; Olshansky, 1962; Richmond, 1973) can indicate the range of reactions. For example, Drotar, Baskiewicz, Irvin, Kennell, and Klaus (1975) elaborated five stages that they found in 25 parents of children with congenital malformations: (1) shock; (2) denial; (3) emotional disequilibrium in which sadness seems to predominate, but anger and anxiety may also occur; (4) adaptation; and (5) reorganization. By using stage theories, therapists can name some of the family members' intense feelings when they have a child with a handicap and put these feelings in a "normal" developmental context. At the same time, the therapist should note that these stages are not necessarily always experienced, nor are they necessarily sequential.

Case Example: Family Reaction

In the vignette that opened this article, the father initially wanted to put the child up for adoption, fearing what the addition of this child would mean to his family or, as his brothers put it, "not wanting a monster in the family." Over time, as the parents had contact with their daughter, learned more about Down's syndrome, and talked to a parent who had raised a Down's syndrome child, they began to view their Zoe as a person with some handicaps, rather than as a case of Down's syndrome.

The therapist who worked with this family focused on (1) respecting and joining their pace, fears, and thoughtfulness in integrating this baby into their life and (2) increasing the ability of the parents to hear and support each other's fears and disappointments. For some time, a pattern had existed in this family in which the mother was afraid to go to the father with negative feelings. The rigidity of this pattern only increased with the birth of the daughter and the mother's guilt about pushing to bring the child home. Positively connoting how the parents balanced and protected each other from difficult issues with this pattern, the therapist helped them to open up their interaction.

Next, the therapist helped family members work through their individual feelings of responsibility for the child's handicap, particularly the mother's thoughts that her body had somehow failed the child. In reviewing all that she had done for the baby as she was pregnant and imagining what she might have done if she had known that the baby had Down's syndrome (i.e., had an abortion), the mother came to a greater acceptance of the baby's condition, realizing that she would not necessarily have intervened to change things, and that she had done everything possible for this child during the pregnancy.

Finally, the therapist helped the parents to continue to plan and follow through on family activities for all five of them, defining the family as a new unit. Over a period of 2 months, the family moved from a frame of "we let you down, child," which emphasized the handicap of the child, to a frame of "we gave you *life,* child," which allowed the family to appreciate the child's potential growth. They began to believe that, if the world came to love E.T., then surely the world would come to love this child.

GUIDELINES FOR THERAPISTS

1. Help families to see all the normal aspects of the child, with the handicap as only one part of the child.
2. When appropriate, share with families the common reactions of similarly situated families (considering onset, time of discovery, type of handicap, etc.).
3. Reassure families that they are the only ones who can make final decisions on care for the child.
4. Use stage theories of reaction cautiously. While they can help to name some of the intense feelings family members are having, the therapist should not implicitly push the family members to move in some sequential order through the stages.
5. Legitimize for families the fact that their range of reactions with a child with a handicap will be the same as that with any child, e.g., anger, frustration, joy. It is OK to be upset with a child with a handicap, as it is OK to be upset with any child from time to time.

DEVELOPMENTAL LIFE CYCLE ISSUES

With the entrance of a baby or young child into any family, there are many rapid developmental shifts (Bradt, 1980). If the baby has a handicap, the adaptations of the family over the first years of life can become more complex.

If there are complications during the pregnancy and birth or adoption procedures, parents may already have fears about the child's well-being. These fears may make it harder for them to prepare themselves and other family members for the arrival of the child. If at birth or on adoption there are clear signs of a problem, parents may keep a certain distance from other new parents. For example, they may not join the usual camaraderie among strangers on a maternity ward. The baby may be in an incubator or need other special medical attention, or the mother may go home while the baby remains in the hospital. Rites of passage around the birth, such as having people come to visit, to hold the baby, and to bring presents, may be affected, because friends and relatives are not sure how they should react. As one father said after his daughter had been born with a rare genetic skin disease,

> My father-in-law was a little scared at first. O.K., he wasn't quite sure how to react. But he, like he was downstairs doing something

when we went over the first time and . . . my mother-in-law went up to see Ianina in the hospital. Dad, my father-in-law didn't, he doesn't like hospitals anyway. So it was no big thing, and when we came to the house Dad was downstairs and I went down and said, "Hi, come on up and see Ianina" and it was, you know, that type of thing. He wasn't waiting at the door. But afterwards it was love at first sight. (Roth, 1983, p. 19)

The family may try not to become too attached to the child for fear that the child will not survive. The entrance of the baby into the family may not be clear-cut as the child goes back and forth to the hospital or the family tries to decide how best to care for the child. This can make it more difficult for the family to reorganize as a larger unit with the addition of another person.

The extensive nurturing and care-giving that all young children need may be complicated by the various medical procedures required. The level of care-giving may also remain higher for a longer time, as the child develops more slowly. The energy and excitement that normally carries new parents forward as their baby becomes more interactive, mobile, and capable of some self-care tasks, such as hold the bottle or finger-feed, may not be as available as a stimulus for the parents or siblings of a child with a handicap. Other milestones, such as walking, talking, dressing, and toilet training, that give parents a sense of movement may also be delayed or may not occur at all. Wikler (1981) identified predictable crises that parents experience as a result of their child's failure to achieve major developmental milestones. Also, as Featherstone (1980) noted, siblings may soon tire of playing with a less responsive child, and more responsibility may fall on the parents to substitute for sibling interaction. Family members may need to find ways to keep supporting and stimulating each other as they nurture the child with special needs.

As families deal daily with variations in developmental functioning, larger issues arise for them. Not only the nuclear family, but also the extended family (Gabel & Kotsch, 1981) and, to some extent, the neighborhood must shift to integrate a new member. This integration may be more problematic if the baby needs extensive care-giving, looks different, or is often in the hospital. Grandparents or other relatives may feel unable to care for the child, may somehow blame themselves for the handicap, or may stay away because it is painful for them to see the child suffering. It may also be more difficult for nuclear family members to maintain contacts with extended family as they go on their rounds of appointments and treatments or as one or both parents work more hours to cover extra costs. As one father described the first year of his premature daughter's life,

> I was working the store probably twelve-fourteen hours a day and the store was not able to pay me enough salary, so I got myself an outside job to get more income, and to get some medical coverage and everything else.
> ... She (my wife) was so busy going, she was in doctors' offices three, four days a week. (Roth, 1983, p. 22)

Family members may withdraw from the neighborhood as they wonder what the neighbors' reactions will be and as the social service network in some ways substitutes for other contacts outside the family. Siblings may not know what to say to playmates about the handicap, or they may stay close to home, sensing the need for help in the house. Hewett (1970) and Hunt (1973) cited complicated care, lack of money, and parental fatigue and embarrassment as factors that curtail family activities outside the home.

As the child with a handicap grows older and has more contact with people outside the home, parents must deal with issues of day care or preschool experiences. Parents may find it difficult to arrange for satisfactory child care, and they may have to reach out to structure or organize peer contact for their child. As the child emerges from the home more, siblings may have to deal with increasing teasing and questioning from other children.

Time and space become precious commodities within the family. Boundaries become less clear-cut for some parts of the outside world (e.g., social service agencies) and perhaps more rigid with others (e.g., neighbors, friends, extended family). The net effect may be less flexible boundaries within the family. Because of the extra care required by the child with a handicap, parents may need to focus on the parental subsystem at the expense of the marital subsystem even more than is usual with young children. Siblings may feel a loss because parents are away from home more. Role divisions around care-giving may become more rigid, as certain skills must be learned specifically for the child with a handicap.

As the family experiences these adjustments, the therapist can help by acknowledging some of these complications of normal developmental issues, while highlighting creative ways in which other families have adapted. Parents and siblings can be placed in contact with other families that have a member with special needs (Park, 1979) so that they can hear and share common problems.

In summary, the therapist should adhere to the following guidelines:

1. Emphasize the normal aspects of the developmental transitions that the family is experiencing.
2. Help the family to see the unique developmental milestones of the child with a handicap.
3. Help to recreate family rituals or passages as seems appropriate (e.g., celebrations around the birth if the family was not able to have the customary celebrations).
4. Place family members in contact with parent groups or sibling groups if desired.
5. Work with social service agencies and the family to minimize stress of additional tasks required by the network or therapeutic programs.
6. Help families with management skills, if needed; direct them to economic, homemaker, and respite support if desired.

LARGER SYSTEMS

In working with families that have a young child with a handicap, the family therapist may want to facilitate a coordinated team approach. It is a rare therapist who is trained in all the services that the family may need in addition to family therapy, such as medical care, physical or educational therapy, information about available resources, and help with day-to-day management skills. Also, the handicap is often not fully understood at this stage, so there is a need for information exchange between the family and "specialists." Although parents are likely to have essential data about their particular child that are not available to anyone else, they are probably still gathering as much information as possible regarding the ramifications of the handicap as the child develops. The family therapist should join them in this and should not consider it a way to avoid the realities of their child's limitations.

It is essential that agencies and the family have a similar view of the role of the family therapist who is working at the interface of larger systems. When referrals are made, the family therapist may be asked to (1) help the family understand the range of family reactions and the impact of the child with special needs on the family, (2) help the family deal with the extra caregiving and stress, (3) help the family obtain services, (4) fill in a gap in services. When relationships between the family and other agencies are problematic, a family therapist may be asked to fix the problem somehow, persuade the family to follow a particular program that an agency is recommending, or handle family-agency frustration that the child is not making as much progress as expected. The family therapist must decide which of these roles are appropriate while, at the same time, determining the place that family therapy may have in the homeostasis of larger systems. As outlined by Coppersmith (1983), problems that may arise when many agencies are working with a family include linear blame of the family for frustrations in the case, overinvolvement of agency personnel with clients, undefined or competing leadership, and dysfunctional agency-family triads.

Work with families in a multidisciplinary approach must be done in a fashion that respects their strengths and does not undermine family capabilities. One of the most important contributions that the family therapist can make to the team is a perspective on the family members' reactions to various treatments and interventions; with this perspective, programs that enhance family interaction can be designed. For instance, if one parent has become involved in a home educational program for the child with special needs to the exclusion of the child's siblings, the therapist may help to plan a program in such a way that some games and activities include all family members, or are self-correcting, so that the siblings can do them alone. In treatment planning, the family therapist should help those involved to question the assumption that "what is good for the child is good for the family" (Doernberg, 1978, p. 107). Particular treatment regimes for a child should be considered within a priority system that takes into account the effect of that regime on the whole family. Doernberg (1978) argued that, occasionally, more treatment for small amelioration of a handicap may not be worth the stress on overall family functioning.

Finally, the family therapist may be required to coordinate the confusion that inevitably arises when the "diagnosis" is uncertain and many people are involved. There are times when various professionals contradict each other, or when the family wants "the answer" and no one is able to frame it in precise terms. The family therapist, in naming confusion as an issue, can help everyone find ways to handle it.

Case example: Larger systems

A mental health service coordinator referred a family for treatment, expressing concern about the parents' adjustment to their son's handicap. John, Jr., age 4, had flaccid paralysis in all limbs and was moderately retarded as a result of cerebral palsy. The service coordinator was worried about the mother's expressed frustrations in having to work with four agencies in order to obtain services for her son, as well as the father's apparent distance from helping professionals and the family.

When the family therapist contacted the family, the mother voiced concerns about a difficult relationship with the service coordinator, and the father said that he thought too many demands were being made on the mother. The family therapist framed her own involvement with the family as entirely voluntary. The parents then invited the therapist to their home for one session. On hearing this from the therapist, the service coordinator invited himself for the session as well. The therapist declined the offer, commenting on all that the coordinator had done to help the family so far and suggesting that he take a break from his efforts. This not only gave the therapist an opportunity to see if the family wanted to engage in treatment, but also marked the boundary between therapy and service coordination.

The parents decided to meet with the therapist over several months, saying that this was the first time that they felt *they* were receiving attention. The parents talked with the therapist about the stress arising from their relationship with outside systems; they had made a major geographical move within the past year, the father was in a more demanding job, and the mother was now far away from her family network of support that had previously helped to transport and care for their son. The parents expressed concern about their isolation, lack of support, the father's being away from home more, and their 5-year-old daughter's changed behavior in that she was more docile and the "good" kid, yet less attentive to her brother.

The therapist framed their concerns within the developmental transitions brought about by all their life changes and worked with them specifically in three areas: (1) increasing the father's involvement with the agencies treating his son, (2) giving the mother more time to be with the daughter, and (3) educating the parents about their rights to solicit and reject services. This pulled the father back into the home, bringing the parents closer together and helping them to work as a team around their son's needs, and gently eliminated the service coordinator's function of "running interference" between the family system and outside systems. Treatment terminated after 4 months. In follow-up a year later, the mother was taking courses part-time, the daughter had made a smooth transition into first grade, the father felt reconnected to the family, and John, Jr. was doing well in a class for children with special needs.

GUIDELINES FOR THERAPISTS

1. Identify all the people and agencies working with a family, and build relationships with them either through a group meeting or individual contacts.

everyone seemed to feel a little bit guilty, like they weren't doing enough for their child. That maybe there is something more or something else that they could be doing to help a little bit more. So there was a lot of certain amount of anxiety over, "Am I doing everything I can?" (Roth, 1983, p. 26)

Gradually, families come to trust their own capabilities. As Featherstone (1980) so eloquently stated:

Fears ease as experience discredits fantasy, as mothers and fathers learn that actual problems of raising their child differ from the ones they had imagined. Similarly, small victories over private demons reassure parents about their own ability to raise their child. (p. 27)

Case example: Family adaptation

A special needs teacher who also had training in family therapy went into the home of one family to work with their daughter Nilda. Her development had been normal until early elementary school, when she went into a coma that lasted 6 months. No specific diagnosis of her resulting disability had ever been established, but her voluntary movements were limited to head turning, eye gazing, utterances of several consonants, and limited oral-motor function. There were two older siblings, and the father worked outside the home.

The teacher took the position that, although the family was not asking for therapy, any interventions that he made with the daughter should be done from a systems perspective that took into account the whole family adaptation. In his assessment, the family was clearly very close and committed to the daughter; however, the siblings were finding it difficult to reconnect with her. Furthermore, there seemed to be a rigidity of roles around the care-giving (i.e., the mother did most of it), and the parents were expressing a need for some help threading their way through the maze of social services.

As the teacher worked to improve Nilda's skills, he tried to address family needs. He taught the two siblings games and activities that they could do with their sister. He adjusted his schedule to be there in the evening when the father was there. At first, the father kept his distance, and the teacher joined with him around various household tasks. Gradually, the father began to watch the exercises being done with Nilda and worked out with his wife a scheduled time when they could work together with Nilda each day after the other two children were sleeping.

2. Gather information about the family's view of this network and the network's view of the family.
3. Clearly define who has what role, e.g., who is in charge of the child's educational needs.
4. Clarify the agencies' view, as well as the family's view, of the role of family therapy: the purpose, time frame, and expectations.
5. Determine how the family interfaces with the social system network and vice versa. Is it helpful or detrimental to long-range family functioning? Define clearly the time line of involvement of all.
6. Coach parents on ways to work with the social system networks that support family strengths by making appointments in evening hours, when more family members are available, and by inviting parents to all treatment planning meetings.

FAMILY ADAPTATION

Over time, the family reorganizes, and its members reach a common understanding of what it means to have a family member with a handicap. If the family is functioning well, the child is defined by many qualities other than the handicap, and the future is believed to encompass growth possibilities for the child and family; the family is realistic about future limitations, however. For instance, a father whose first child was born with spina bifida had known that the baby was a boy since 5 months before his birth. During the pregnancy, he had visions of father-son tennis doubles some day. After the birth, as he put it, "I had to give up that idea. Since then I've realized there's a lot of other things he can do and there are other things I can teach him." The father now envisions sitting down with the boy at the computer terminal and teaching him about computers.

The family structure also must be reorganized in such a way that no one person carries the burden of all the extra day-to-day work that having a child with a handicap may entail, both inside and outside the home. All family members must have sources of renewal and energy. At the same time, the structure must be flexible enough to accommodate the range of issues that will arise in the future. For instance, families may have to deal with more cycles of ambiguity, i.e., not knowing the meaning of new developments, trying to gather new information, and incorporating new situations into family functioning. In addition, families may feel that they should be doing more to help the child. As one father described parents who had young children with a handicap in his support group,

As part of his tutoring, the teacher taught the parents to act as advocates for their daughter, advising them on services, legislation, and their rights. After 6 months, both parents were fully participating in Nilda's program. The father was making direct contact with social service agencies, including hosting the teacher when the mother had to be away from home; the siblings had found more ways to be with Nilda; and the parents were more assertive regarding services for their daughter.

GUIDELINES FOR THERAPISTS

1. Reassure them that there is no right or wrong way for a family to organize itself in response to a handicap.
2. Acknowledge that some issues may always be with family members in some way, such as (a) feelings that they are not doing enough for the child, (b) more complex life cycle transitions, (c) cycles of ambiguity and readjustment.
3. To protect the family system, teach family members about their rights and expectations of those who "help" them.
4. Help family members to assess the way in which their day-to-day family organization supports and works for them with their extra responsibilities for the child with special needs.
5. Bring in the future time frame so that families consider what they expect life to be like in 5 years with their child with a handicap, 10 years, etc.

CONCLUSION

The guidelines offered here can be useful not only for family therapists, but also for people who are working with families in their homes to provide services for the child with special needs. These guidelines are intended only as general parameters. Each family's individual experiences must be respected. Families can be functional and healthy in the face of often extraordinary pressures. The more I talk and work with families, the more I appreciate their strengths and their willingness to share and teach therapists about the variety of possible ways to be in the world.

Acknowledgments: I am indebted to Sanford Roth, M.Ed., Deborah Saperstone, MSW, and Jeff Green, Ph.D., for their contributions of case materials and to Susan Hawes and Noor-Anisa Bodin for their research assistance.

REFERENCES

Barsch, R.H. (1968). *The parent of the handicapped child: Study of child rearing practices.* Springfield, IL: Charles C. Thomas.

Baum, M.H. (1962). Some dynamic factors affecting family adjustment to the handicapped child. *Exceptional Child, 28,* 387–392.

Bradt, J.O. (1980). The family with young children. In E. Carter & M. McGoldrick (Eds.), *The family life cycle: A framework for family therapy.* New York: Gardner Press.

Coppersmith, E. (1983). The place of family therapy in the homeostasis of larger systems. In M. Aronson & R. Wolberg (Eds.), *Group and family therapy, 1982: An overview.* New York: Brunner Mazel.

Doernberg, N. (1978). Some negative effects on family integration of health and educational services for young handicapped children. *Rehabilitation Literature, 39*(4), 107–110.

Drotar, D., Baskiewicz, A., Irvin, N., Kennell, J., & Klaus, M. (1975). The adaptation of parents to the birth of an infant with a congenital malformation: A hypothetical model. *Pediatrics, 56,* 710–716.

Falicov, C.J. (1983). *Cultural perspectives in family therapy.* Rockville, MD: Aspen Systems Corporation.

Farber, B. (1960). Perceptions of crisis and related variables in the impact of a retarded child on the mother. *Journal of Health and Human Behavior, 1,* 108–118.

Featherstone, H. (1980). *A difference in the family.* New York: Basic Books.

Fotheringham, J.B., & Cereal, D. (1974). Handicapped children and handicapped families. *International Review of Education, 20*(3), 355–373.

Gabel, H., & Kotsch, L.S. (1981). Extended families and young handicapped children. *Topics in Early Childhood Special Education, 1,* 29–35.

Gayton, W.F., Friedman, S.B., Tavormina, J.F., & Tucker, F. (1977). Children with cystic fibrosis: 1. Psychological test findings of patients, siblings and parents. *Pediatrics, 59,* 888–894.

Hewett, S. (1970). *The family and the handicapped child: A study of cerebral palsied children in their homes.* Chicago: Aldine.

Holroyd, J. (1974). The questionnaire on resources and stress: An instrument to measure family response to a handicapped member. *Journal of Community Psychology, 2,* 92–94.

Holroyd, J., Brown, N., Wikler, L., & Simmons, J.Q. (1975). Stress in families of institutionalized and noninstitutionalized autistic children. *Journal of Community Psychology, 3,* 26–31.

Howell, S.E. (1973). Psychiatric aspects of habilitation. *Pediatric Clinics of North America, 20,* 203–219.

Hunt, G.M. (1973). Implications of the treatment of myelomeningocele for the child and the family. *Lancet, 2,* 1308.

Klaus, M., & Kennell, J. (1976). *Maternal-infant bonding.* St. Louis: C.V. Mosby.

McAllister, R.J., Butler, E., & Lei, T.J. (1973). Patterns of social interaction among families of behaviorally retarded children. *Journal of Marriage and the Family, 35,* 93–100.

McGoldrick, M., Pearce, J.K., & Giordano, J. (Eds.). (1982). *Ethnicity and family therapy.* New York: Guilford Press.

Murphy, M. (1982). The family with a handicapped child: A review of the literature. *Journal of Behavioral and Developmental Pediatrics, 3*(2), 73–82.

Olshansky, S. (1962). Chronic sorrow: A response to having a mentally defective child. *Social Casework, 43,* 190–194.

Park, L.D. (1979). The summer family conference: An adventure in counseling families with handicapped children. *Rehabilitation Literature, 40*(4), 108–110.

Richmond, J.B. (1973). The family and the handicapped child. *Clinical Proceedings, 29*(7), 156–164.

Roskies, E. (1972). *Abnormality and normality: The mothering of thalidomide children.* Ithaca, NY: Cornell University Press.

Roth, S. (1983). [Unpublished transcripts, University of Massachusetts at Amherst].

Sheridan, M. (1965). *The handicapped child and his home.* London: National Childrens Homes.

Sultz, H.A., Schlesinger, E.R., Mosher, W.E., & Feldman, J.G. (1972). *Long-term childhood illness.* Pittsburgh: University of Pittsburgh Press.

Tropauer, A., Franz, M.N., & Delgard, V.W. (1970). Psychological aspects of the care of children with cystic fibrosis. *American Journal of Diseases of Children, 119,* 424–432.

Turk, J. (1964). Impact of cystic fibrosis on family functioning. *Pediatrics, 34,* 67–71.

Weber, G., & Parker, T. (1981). A study of family and professional views of the factors affecting family adaptation to a disabled child. In N. Stinnett, J. DeFrain, K. King, P. Knaub, & G. Rowe (Eds.), *Family strengths 3: Roots of well-being.* Omaha: University of Nebraska Press.

Wikler, L. (1981). Chronic stresses of families of mentally retarded children. *Family Relations, 30,* 281–288.

Wikler, L., Wasow, M., & Hatfield, E. (1981). Chronic sorrow revisited: Parent vs. professional depiction of the adjustment of parents of mentally retarded children. *American Journal of Orthopsychiatry, 51,* 63–70.

Zisserman, L. (1981). The modern family and rehabilitation of the handicapped: A macrosociological view. *American Journal of Occupational Therapy, 35*(1), 13–20.

2. Working with Families of School-Aged Handicapped Children

Lee Combrinck-Graham
L. Wayne Higley

School-Aged Handicapped Children 19

THE PROBLEMS FACED BY FAMILIES WITH SCHOOL-AGED HANDICAPPED children are different from those faced by families with younger handicapped children. The developmental issues that affect the families of children whose handicaps are identified after they enter school can be similar to those that affect the families of "longitudinally" handicapped children (i.e., children with physical, intellectual, social, and emotional handicaps that are recognized before school entry), however. Although the problems of handicapped youngsters in school have been addressed in volumes of material in the mental health and education literature, the particular problems of the *families* of the handicapped during the school years are only now being investigated.

FAMILY LIFE CYCLE

Family structure oscillates from centripetal to centrifugal states through the life spiral (Combrinck-Graham, 1983). Children reach school age at a point in the family life cycle when the family is moving away from the intense centripetal organization that surrounded the children's births and early childhood. In the course of normal family evolution, the family that has been relatively self-contained and somewhat immune to outside influences becomes vulnerable to the scrutiny of the world outside its home when the children go to school. Ordinarily, the exchange between the family system and its external environment becomes greater. In healthy families, this exchange facilitates the appropriate differentiation of the individuals in the family during the centrifugal period, when the children are adolescent. In families with handicapped children, however, these processes are altered in several ways.

First, the recognition of the handicap usually results in an exchange between family members and outside professionals at an earlier stage. The family may annex professionals by integrating their support and advice into its way of being together. In effect, the family is not an autonomous, self-contained group and, perhaps, forfeits the development of a secure base of intimacy from which differentiation usually takes place.

Second, the needs of the handicapped child may interfere with the "normal" differentiating process. The healthy exchange that usually results from the child's coming and going may be tempered by a parent's coming and going with the child. Thus, the unit of parent(s) and child may remain intact, preventing both the child and the parent(s) from having their more differentiated experiences outside the family. If the child has been involved in the highly personalized experience of special treatment or educational settings during the preschool period, the parents may find the bureaucratic maze of the school system overwhelming. Although P.L. 94–142 mandates education tailored to the special needs of each handicapped student, parents must often find their own way through school system labyrinths to locate helpful personnel and programs suitable for their children. Since the parents are not experts in diagnosis or education, this effort can be stressful, as is detailed in an increasing literature on the parent and P.L. 94–142 (Strickland, 1983).

Unless their handicapping condition is so severe that they are unaware of their surroundings, handicapped children are bound to become more aware of their difference when exposed to the school environment. Similarly, siblings become more aware of the difference and, therefore, their own difference. These differences are accentuated by the natural self-comparison and the effort to be as "good" as peers that characterize the social organization of school-age children (Minuchin, 1977). Difference is particularly painful to school-aged children, since their awareness is not tempered with understanding. Featherstone (1980) reported the results of a study in which handicapped youngsters were asked about their feelings about mainstreaming. Those who felt very different from other children preferred to be in separate classes, showing a desire to retreat from the normal social environment of the school-aged child.

For the parents, there is also more exposure and, possibly, more shame when their handicapped child enters school. Parents who have been most active in seeking diagnosis and therapy for their child in the preschool period have usually found some solace among the professionals and other parents with whom they have worked. Although these kinds of relationships may be renewed or continued in a special education setting, there is less protection in these settings. Parents who have been less involved with their child's handicap are even more vulnerable. While other children are solving the mysteries of reading and math, mastering their worlds by learning about current events and history, unlocking the secrets of science, developing their bodies into well-calibrated instruments, the handicapped child is occupied in learning less singular skills. Their unfulfilled expectations may explain the observation that parents of school-aged handicapped children experience chronic sorrow or recurrent grief (Wikler, 1981; Wikler, Wasow, & Hatfield, 1981). Long after it would be expected that they "should have adjusted" to their child's handicap, the parents experience a renewed sense of loss, clearly connected with the achievements of each developmental stage that their child cannot attain.

FAMILY PATTERNS

Although there are virtually no studies on the structure of families with school-aged handicapped youngsters, there appear to be some characteristic patterns of organization in these families. Foster and Berger (1979) and Berger (1982) observed that some characteristic structural patterns in families with handicapped preschoolers become fixed (rigid), thus restricting the families' behavioral repertoires. Following the model presented by Minuchin, Rosman, and Baker (1978) for psychosomatic families, Foster and Berger illustrated three dysfunctional structural patterns that may occur in families of handicapped preschoolers: (1) a rigid three-generational triad, (2) a scapegoating pattern, and (3) a stable condition involving the child with one parent.

Perosa (1980) looked for specific characteristics of psychosomatic families in the families of learning-disabled youngsters. Assessing enmeshment and conflict resolution, Perosa found that the families of the learning-disabled youngsters were not generally enmeshed. One parent, usually the father, was often distinctly disengaged, while the mother and child were overinvolved with one another. On the other hand, conflict resolution in these families was poor, and the learning-disabled child tended to become involved in conflicts between the parents, much as described by Minuchin and associates. Featherstone (1980) observed that the presence of a handicapped child threatens important boundaries in the family, both within the family and at its border. She described the handicapped child as outside the sibling system and in danger of encroaching on the parent system. Furthermore, she remarked on the influence of professionals on the family's home life, confirming the notion that the family system expands in some way to include the professionals.

A dysfunctional pattern in a family system may be replicated in the family-school interaction (Coppersmith, 1982). The school may increase the father's disengagement by accepting the mother as the representative of the "family." This increases the mother's expertise and involvement with the child, while the father may become even more disengaged. In other instances, the parents may unite against the school, viewing the experts as demeaning, critical, or simply not helpful; this creates a process of mutual blame that is perpetuated until one side surrenders. Rubin and Quinn-Curan (1983) recommended that the school experts acknowledge the parents' continuing sensitivity and the importance of keeping alive the hope that the child will be able to accomplish more. In this spirit, the experts can support the parents.

ROLE OF FAMILY THERAPY

When parents ask for help with any aspect of the management of their handicapped child, they provide an opportunity to assess not only the child, but also the systems around the child. Included are intrafamilial patterns, such as the way in which the family as a system and its individual members are coping with current developmental issues, and the family's relations with extrafamilial contacts that involve the child. There is a natural resistance to this, because the presence of a clearly defined handicapping condition is, to the family, obviously "the problem." The handicap may have been confirmed by the school through placement in a special class and development of an Individualized Education Program (IEP). The family may have undergone a great deal of agony and stress to arrive at the delicate balance between acceptance of the handicap and hope for improvement. They may be reluctant to allow anyone to tamper with their delicately balanced system.

The child's entry into school usually requires the family to adjust to new personnel and to their rules and rituals. Just as school can be an experience that increases the child's independence of the family and the parents' independence of the child, it places new expectations on the family system, requiring change. School personnel expect progress in the child, but they do not always understand that this must be associated with change in the family. Rarely does the school make any comprehensive effort to help the family make these changes.

In most cases, the family is referred for outside help because school personnel feel that the handicapped child is not developing as predicted; this usually means that the child or the parents are not behaving as school personnel think they should. Although these families need to be more inventive than families who do not have a handicapped child, they are less willing to upset the patterns of family life, with all the stress that such a disruption entails. They believe that they must protect the rules, roles, and relationships that have been established and have become familiar and comfortable in the home. Thus, what may be perceived as uncooperative behavior may actually be the family's efforts to maintain their hard-won equilibrium.

Family-School Interaction

Coppersmith (1982) observed that there are both advantages and disadvantages to family therapy within the school system. Offering family therapy through the school does make it possible to coordinate the family-school interface. Without this coordination, school personnel may blame the family environment for the difficulties that they experience with the child in school, or they may take the child's side against the family. Working together, school personnel and family members can seek new solutions to problems that have traditionally been handled by sending the child to the principal or the nurse, or on other routes by which the attempted solution becomes the problem.

When the therapy is undertaken in the school, however, roles should be clearly defined. Parents cannot be therapists, nor can teachers. When a child is having difficulties in school, the system needing intervention includes both the family and the educational personnel. The family therapist/consultant should be familiar with school procedures and personnel, but should not be directly involved in the educational process. Appropriately trained school counselors could function in this role *if* they have enough independence from the school's administrative structure to make interventions in school structures. The therapist can enter the family-school system either through the family or through the school, or may work with both simultaneously.

The family consultant can influence the family system through the school. For example, in one special school where there was a strong commitment to working with parents, the requirement of weekly half-hour parent involvement sessions was generally met by a meeting between the teacher and the mother, often without the child. Through work with a consultant, the staff became increasingly aware of family issues, such as disagreements between parents about the best way to handle the child, or an excessive burden on one parent accentuated by the lack of involvement of the other. They felt obligated to confine their interventions to educational tasks, however, and did not include a family evaluation as part of their initial assessment, acceptance, or goal-setting procedures. Consequently, when they became aware of family dysfunction after working with a child, it seemed to them that their entrance into the family system would be considered an invasion and would be met with resistance. The consultant was able to help them use their observations about the families by including other family members in "parent involvement" sessions, thus keeping the educational focus, but involving the families in a way that could effect useful change for them. A future goal for this school system is to include a family assessment in the admission process so that family and educational issues can be blended. Family members can then carry out educational processes at home, while the teachers can support effective family functioning in working with the child at school.

The consultant to a school about families may also need to be a consultant to families about schools, and we developed a workshop for families on how to "conduct" a parent-teacher meeting. The object of the workshop was to help parents see themselves as experts on the child in one area meeting experts on the child in another area in order to develop a complementary relationship in the total care of the child. At the workshop, teachers were available so that parents could "practice." As the parents were invited to present themselves as experts, the teachers were invited to use the parents as consultants. For example, one of the teachers asked a parent about a problem that she, the teacher, had with the child's behavior at mealtimes. The parent reported that the behavior in question was unacceptable at home, and the child was required to eat by himself when he did it. She suggested that the teacher do the same at school. This kind of interaction had never occurred at a previous parent-teacher meeting.

Families in Family Therapy

There is a role for a family therapist in each of the problem areas that have been discussed. In one family, for example, a developmental issue pressed on a family system that had functioned well (although not painlessly) until the "normal" child's approach to adolescence placed new demands on her relationship with her mother.

Case Example

> Bonnie and Mel were parents of a retarded 9-year-old, Jim, and a bright, vivacious 12-year-old, Melanie. Bonnie had spent most of her time in the past 3 years obtaining a proper school placement for Jim; at the time of the consultation, things were going well for him. They had asked for the consultation because they were not sure how to deal with a serious conflict between Melanie and her mother, who were fighting constantly. Melanie had threatened to leave home, and Bonnie was angry and frightened. Mel had much less trouble with Melanie, who, he thought, accepted his authority and did not draw him into the battles of will that she had with her mother.
> Mel resisted a family consultation because he felt that the problem was Bonnie's. He felt that Bonnie needed help for herself with a chance to look at her life and think about her own goals. She was a smart, well-educated woman who had neglected her own personal and professional growth to concentrate on Jim. Mel reasoned that, if Bonnie were happier and clearer about her own goals, she would be able to interact more

effectively with Melanie. He finally agreed to a family consultation because he loved his wife and wanted to help her.

In the interview, Mel took some time to describe the family history over the previous 9 years. As he and Bonnie began to recognize that Jim was different, Mel went into "3-year shock." He felt guilty that he left all the efforts to determine what was the matter with Jim to his wife. He often wept alone in the night, sorry for Jim, for his wife, and for himself, but put on a front for Bonnie. He felt grateful to Bonnie for dealing with all aspects of this stressful period. As he began to be more at peace with the family situation, his business began to fail; for several years, his time was consumed in managing a bankruptcy and subsequent reorganization. For the past 2 years, he had been preoccupied with making his business work and was now beginning to feel somewhat successful.

A pattern had developed. Bonnie was the expert care-giver for Jim; Mel was removed not only from issues in Jim's management, but also from Bonnie. Consequently, Mel felt that he had been unavailable to Bonnie during some critical times, but he did not associate this with his identification of her current needs, which he felt should be met by individual therapy. He could agree, however, that he would have to be involved if her first priority were to improve her relationship with Melanie. Encouraged by the therapist, she asserted that such improvement was indeed her first priority, and they agreed to family therapy.

In actuality, both the mother and the daughter were facing a similar challenge—to become more independent. This challenge arose in the context of a hard-won and successful struggle to get Jim settled in the appropriate environment. The needs of all the other family members had been somewhat neglected in the family's concern for Jim. Melanie's bid for some attention to her development was, at first, met with irritation by her mother, who was ill-prepared to deal with demands from her "whole" child. Mel had become the "disengaged father," and he would probably have continued in that role if Bonnie had received individual treatment.

While the family, with Mel's voice, was initially resistant to an approach that threatened the family's adjustment to Jim's handicapping condition, the consultation presented an opportunity to deal with key issues for the family, such as Mel's availability to Bonnie and Bonnie's availability to Melanie, and to investigate new ways of organizing that would increase the satisfaction of all the family members.

Mel and Bonnie's family conformed to a very common structural pattern in families with handicapped children: the mother focused on the management of the handicapped child, the father preoccupied with other issues, and the sibling(s) relatively underparented. Marital issues were not addressed directly and, in fact were put aside, indefinitely postponed, or not even recognized. The focal point was the attention to the handicapped child's needs. Melanie's challenge, in this case, brought the opportunity for a new perspective for the family.

The second case also illustrates a family's loss of contact with important issues involving family members other than the handicapped youngster. In this case, the parents sacrificed themselves and their relationship to care for their children. The nonhandicapped siblings had made their own ways in the family by being extremely demanding, thus further depleting the parent system. The case was sent to family therapy at the recommendation of the handicapped child's teacher, who felt that there was a significance to the child's destructive behavior, although she could not define it. The treatment involved several family-school meetings.

Case Example

> Louise and Don sought therapy because their 12-year-old brain-damaged, adopted son, Danny, was becoming almost impossible to manage. Impulsive and unpredictable, he often destroyed his own cherished possessions and seemed to have "no sense of connection between cause and effect." Don thought he would have a heart attack during one of the angry sermons in which he attempted to make Danny understand what he was doing. Louise was reduced to banishing Danny to his room almost nightly. They referred to his behavior as his "shtick," an inevitable characteristic. Initial sessions included the parents; Danny; his chubby 9-year-old sister, Amanda, who was verbal, demanding, and unpopular with her peers; and another sister, Jane, a college freshman who was having difficulty with her roommate and demanded that her father make the 3-hour trip each way to pick her up and return her to college every weekend.
>
> A turning point in treatment came when a family session was held at Danny's school so that his teacher could participate. Earlier, the teacher had agreed to send home weekly reports of Danny's school troubles, not realizing that these reports confirmed the parents' conviction that Danny was not able to control himself. Citing the fact that he recorded the anger and unfairness he felt about his younger sister in a daily diary at school, the teacher expressed the belief that Danny knew what he was doing. Jane agreed with the teacher. As Danny's feelings about Amanda were clarified, his father agreed that she was spoiled, provocative, and overprotected. At this point, the family structure had shifted around the intervention of the teacher, since the teacher, the father, and Danny challenged some of the family's habitual patterns of behavior with respect to the children. Danny cried when the therapist wondered about

his fear of being "unadopted," further demonstrating that he was a sensitive, responsive person.

The immediate aftereffect of this session was a change in the teacher's reports to the parents, which now emphasized his awareness and comprehension of his problems. Some changes in disciplinary procedures did end Danny's self-destructive behavior, but not his angry assaults on his family and peers, which became more clearly intentional. As therapy continued and Danny's anger and destructiveness were more clearly connected with family issues and feelings, the teacher could see progress and, thus, was able to tolerate his behavior better. Gradually, as his behavior in school improved, the therapy focused primarily on the family.

It also emerged in early sessions that Louise and Don had almost no private life. Don's work schedule was constantly changing at the whim of his employer (to Louise's disgust). The parents could not leave Danny with a babysitter; he had driven off a series of them. Their older daughter consumed their weekends. Amanda's troubles with her playmates required frequent interventions. In fact, these parents had accepted the tyranny of all their children, not just the handicapped one, at the expense of their adult private life.

Only after some months of treatment did the parents begin to demand that their older daughter make her own weekend plans. Don told Louise about his annoyance with Amanda. In sessions without the children, they discussed the husband's hopes for his wife, which had remained vague, and her need for his help in financial procedures. They began to plan more social activities outside the home and set aside time to be together after the children were in bed. At times, they returned to their youthful dreams about a life together with tearful poignancy. They recognized that, while Danny would continue to be "a handful," they needed and had a right to their own life together.

Clearly, a family systems approach permits the therapist to assess and intervene in a child's problems at a variety of different levels. Both family and school personnel acknowledged that Danny was a problem, and this status was maintained by the teacher's weekly reports, even though the teacher did not actually view the boy's problems as the parents did. At the family level, the boy's difficulties were a part of the burden placed on the parents by all their children, a burden under which they felt helpless. A teacher-family meeting introduced the parents to their child as a feeling individual, changed the nature of the teacher-parent interaction, and initiated an altered pattern within the family that led the parents to reassess their catering to the children at the expense of their own relationship.

Because of the importance of the family's relationship with the school, a consultant must sometimes be willing to challenge both systems.

Case Example

> Malvena had been the sole parent of five children, three of whom were handicapped, since her husband left 10 years ago. Martin, her 10-year-old blind, retarded son was arriving at school almost daily with more money than he should have had and using it to treat his friends. Contacted each time by the principal, Malvena had tried several different techniques to prevent Martin from taking money. She accepted the responsibility, as was her wont, but was almost surprised by her anger not only with Martin, but also with the school personnel, who had always seen her as the model parent. She felt guilty about the fact that during the last 3 years she had gone from volunteer to paid full-time work as a parent advocate at the Association for Retarded Citizens. The calls from the principal interrupted her work almost daily. With support from a consulting family therapist, Malvena *demanded* that the school deal with Martin's "money problems."
>
> The principal knew the family quite well and understood the situation. A procedure was developed at the school for confiscating the money, punishing Martin, and directing him to take the money home. The principal accepted this responsibility because Malvena helped her to understand that it was necessary to deal with the mother and the son as separate and independent individuals.

The difficulty in Malvena's family arose in the context of Malvena's own differentiation into her work. The intervention encouraged a normal family adjustment to a child's school-aged years in which the parents can expect the child to have a meaningful and separate experience at school, while the other family members become involved in their own activities. The agreement between Malvena and the principal not only allowed Malvena to pursue her work, but also held Martin responsible in a social context outside his family.

CONCLUSION

The family therapist has a major function when a handicapped child enters school. The therapist not only can provide therapy in a traditional setting, but also can help families to use their own resources effectively and can help schools to assess family resources in planning and carrying out educational plans for the child.

REFERENCES

Berger, M. (1982). Predictable tasks in therapy with families of handicapped persons. In A.S. Gurman (Ed.), *Questions and answers in the practice of family therapy* (Vol. 2, pp. 82–87). New York: Brunner/Mazel.

Combrinck-Graham, L. (1983). The family life cycle and families with young children. In H. Liddle (Ed.), *The family life cycle*. Rockville, MD: Aspen Systems Corporation.

Coppersmith, E.I. (1982). Family therapy in a public school system. In A.S. Gurman (Ed.), *Questions and answers in the practice of family therapy* (Vol. 2, pp. 268–271). New York: Brunner/Mazel.

Darling, R.B. (1983). Parent-professional interaction: The roots of misunderstanding. In M. Seligman (Ed.), *The family with a handicapped child* (pp. 95–121). New York: Grune and Stratton.

Featherstone, H. (1980). *A difference in the family*. New York: Basic.

Foster, M.A., & Berger, M. (1979). Structural family therapy: Applications in programs for preschool handicapped children. *Journal of the Division of Early Childhood, 1*, 52–58.

Minuchin, P. (1977). *The middle years of childhood*. Monterrey, CA: Brooks/Cole.

Minuchin, S., Rosman, B.L., & Baker, L. (1978). *Psychosomatic families: Anorexia nervosa in context*. Cambridge, MA: Harvard University Press.

Perosa, L.M. (1980). The development of a questionnaire to measure Minuchin's structural family concepts and the application of his psychosomatic family model to learning disabled families. *Dissertation Abstracts, 41A*, 110.

Rubin, S., & Quinn-Curran, N. (1983). Lost, then found: The parents' journey through the community service maze. In M. Seligman (Ed.), *The family with a handicapped child* (pp. 63–94). New York: Grune and Stratton.

Strickland, B. (1983). Legal issues that affect parents. In M. Seligman (Ed.), *The family with a handicapped child* (pp. 27–59). New York: Grune and Stratton.

Wikler, L. (1981). Family therapy with families of mentally retarded children. In A.S. Gurman (Ed.), *Questions and answers in the practice of family therapy* (Vol. 1, pp. 129–132). New York: Brunner/Mazel.

Wikler, L., Wasow, M., & Hatfield, E. (1981). Chronic sorrow revisited: Parent versus professional depiction of the adjustment of parents of mentally retarded children. *American Journal of Orthopsychiatry, 51*, 63–70.

3. From Home to College, From College to Home: An Interactional Approach to Treating the Symptomatic Disabled College Student

Richard A. Whiting
Linda L. Terry
Helyn Strom-Henriksen

LEAVING HOME AND ESTABLISHING A SUCCESSFUL INDEPENDENT LIVing situation is often the primary goal of disabled young adults. Increasingly, higher education is the means for achieving this end, representing the leaving home stage of family development for families with a disabled member. Although it is currently impossible to determine the exact number of disabled college students, Wulfsberg (1980) estimated that 57,700 disabled students were enrolled in U.S. colleges or universities in the fall of 1978. During the last 5 years, there has been a significant increase in the number of disabled students on our campus, and we assume that this is also true at other types of postsecondary institutions. As educational programs have developed at the elementary and secondary levels, more disabled individuals want a college experience to continue their educational and professional development. Without question, the Rehabilitation Act of 1973 and the subsequent federal regulations issued in 1977 have had a positive impact on educational opportunities for the disabled.

TRADITIONAL PERSPECTIVE

The field of rehabilitation has changed dramatically since the early 1900s. At the turn of the century, the emphasis was on custodial care. Today, rehabilitation is considered a dynamic, holistic process designed to help the individual reach the fullest possible level of functioning through comprehensive, ongoing evaluations of specific abilities, limitations, and needs (Goldenson, 1978). Services, which are provided in vocational, educational, social, physical, and psychological areas, are individually oriented. It is assumed that, through self-acceptance, the disabled person can be competent and, if at all possible, self-sufficient. The ultimate goal, which is similar to self-actualization, is to achieve a level of stigma incorporation, a "state in which the fact of the individual's stigmatized condition becomes an integral part of both the majority of the components of the self state as well as the total self state" (DeLoach & Greer, 1981, p. 221). Those who advocate use of the traditional rehabilitation model believe that disabled people leave home when they feel confident or assertive enough to defy their parents (Nigro, 1977).

With such an emphasis on self-acceptance and psychodynamic theory, it is not surprising that the family and the disabled member have traditionally been treated separately, especially during adolescence, the time of independence. Most studies of families with a disabled member have dealt primarily with families of infants and young children, however, emphasizing mother-child interactions (Stanhope & Bell, 1981).

In the traditional rehabilitation process, the goal is to educate and train the parents to cope with and respond to their disabled child. Often, this is done in groups of parents so that parents who have similar difficulties can provide mutual support. For example, there are parent groups for those with children who have such disabilities as mental retardation, spina bifida, or cerebral palsy (Dunham, 1978). Individual or group therapy is also used to facilitate a discussion of parents' attitudes about themselves and their child and, as Briard (1976) suggested, "to help the parents form more realistic expectations and to communicate those to the child" (p. 585). Through such efforts, it is hoped that those with congenital disabilities will, by late adolescence, become sufficiently outgoing to establish and maintain social contacts, sufficiently resilient emotionally to recover from inevitable slights and rejections, and sufficiently astute socially to detect those occasions when their advances are not well received and modify their behavior to increase their chances for success (DeLoach & Greer, 1981).

AN INTERACTIONAL APPROACH

The Disabled

From the traditional perspective, a disability "happens" to an individual and requires adjustment and adaptation by the individual. The behaviors of the family are additive factors, being relevant only to the extent that they support or hinder the disabled family member's progress. Over the past 30 years, therapists working with families of the handicapped have focused on supportive and hindering organizational structures (Haley, 1976; Minuchin, 1974) rather than on individuals' intrapsychic processes. Those who support an interactional approach, however, hold that behavior has meaning only within an interpersonal context and is a response to that context (Jackson, 1967). In this view, there are no causative behaviors that lead to single outcomes. There is only mutual causality, a process in which event A triggers event B, which triggers event C, which triggers event A. The behaviors form a circular, repetitive sequence, the beginning and end of which can be only arbitrarily punctuated. Therefore, the therapist shifts from seeing only the identified patient to working with families, and from searching for and educating the patient on historical and root causes of the problem to identifying and intervening in current problematic interactional sequences of the family.

The pioneering work of Minuchin and his colleagues (1978) with diabetics whose disease was uncontrolled revealed recurring patterns of acidosis and hospitalization when conflict between these patients and their parents was intensified. This observation provided the impetus for the development of a systemic model for understanding psychosomatic disorders. From this research, Minuchin and associates characterized psychosomatic families as enmeshed, overprotective of each other, inflexible, and poor at conflict resolution, particularly in the marital dyad.

While Minuchin and his colleagues classified uncontrolled diabetes and severe asthma as psychosomatic disorders, these problems also qualify as lifelong disabilities that are physically inhibiting, require special care, arouse understandable concern in family members, and have the potential for organizing family members and others around them. Therefore, it makes sense to examine disability from an interactional perspective. Published research on the application of a family systems approach to therapy with families with a physically disabled member is quite scanty, but there have been a few attempts at conceptualizing treatment from a systemic perspective (deParra, 1982; Peck, 1974). A few case examples have demonstrated promising outcomes (Ritterman, 1982; Shapiro & Harris, 1976; Teismann & Rodgers, 1982; Webb-Woodard & Woodard, 1982). In these case examples, with the exception of that described by Webb-Woodard and Woodard, the condition of the disabled individual is viewed as given and static, and the task of the therapist is to guide the family to new management techniques. Neither the fluctuations in the intensity and ability to cope with the disability in response to family interactional patterns, nor the developmental stage of the family life cycle is considered, however.

Family Systems Therapy

Central to family systems therapy is the assumption that problems arise at transitional stages of the family developmental life cycle (Haley, 1973; Minuchin, 1974). The family, not the individual, is the focus of assessment and intervention in therapy. Changes in one individual affect the other members and call for a functional reorganization of the family. If a family does not make the changes necessary to accommodate the accomplishment of a new set of developmental tasks, a problem emerges.

Transitional stages that involve the arrival or departure of a new member have been cited as the most difficult (Haley, 1980). Haley's work on the leaving home stage remains the most thorough in the field on this phase of the family life cycle examined from an interactional perspective. Leaving home to pursue the future is the developmental task of late adolescence. Whether that future includes work, education, or marriage and whether it occurs at age 18 or 30 varies from family to family, but "a young person's success or failure at that task is an inextricable part of the reorganization of a family, as new hierarchical arrangements are made and new communication pathways develop" (Haley, 1980, p. 30). Failure outside the home by the launched child, such as withdrawal from college as a first-semester freshman, may help to maintain stability in a family that is not ready to reorganize (Whiting, 1980). Typically, this occurs when the marital couple cannot address the changes that must be made between them and the difficulties of the child provide a means of communication for the couple. In this case, the goals of therapy are to unite the parents in their efforts to launch the child.

Conceptual Integration

When a disabled young adult who has previously accomplished certain tasks begins to perform incompetently and to increase the involvement of family and others in his or her survival at the leaving home stage of the family life cycle, the regressive behavior may stabilize the family. The open systems model of Minuchin, Rosman, and Baker (1978) illustrates the interactional process of the disability and family functioning (Figure 3–1). In this circular model, a change in any one of the components precipitates a response in another component. Extrafamilial or intrafamilial stress (e.g., denied or unresolved conflict between two members) engages the susceptible child through mediating mechanisms (physiological responses) that precipitate a symptomatic behavior in the child, engaging the family through periodic vascillations in the condition. When the child is away at school,

Figure 3–1 Open Systems Model of Families with a Disabled Member

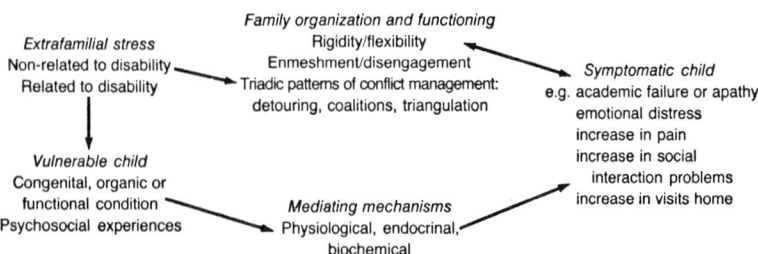

Source: Reprinted by permission from *Psychosomatic Families* by S. Minuchin, B. Rosman, and L. Baker. Cambridge: Harvard University Press, 1978.

however, more extreme noncoping responses may be needed to engage the family. Exacerbations of the disabling condition that require frequent visits home to the long-involved physicians, loss of interest in academic and career goals that results in poor grades, and depression that confirms the family's belief in the child's need for protection perpetuate the homeostatic cycle.

CHARACTERISTICS OF FAMILIES WITH A SYMPTOMATIC DISABLED MEMBER

Our experience over the past 5 years has indicated that families with a disabled college-aged child have certain characteristics in common. These characteristics can be examined in relation to the three dimensions Minuchin used to assess family functioning: degree of disengagement versus enmeshment across boundaries, triadic patterns of conflict management, and ability to adapt to change.

Disengagement vs. Enmeshment

Families with a disabled college-aged adolescent are characterized by extremes of both disengagement and enmeshment. Disengagement may be reflected by an inappropriate denial that the child is doing anything special by attending college and that the child's difficulties are any different from those of other college students. The impact of the disability on the child's social life with peers, sexual development, and opportunities for a traditional future, including marriage, may never be openly acknowledged. Enmeshment may be reflected in the reverberations of the child's fluctuating affective responses throughout the family system. The student's disappointment and frustration may engage the parents in lengthy discussions to convey reassurance and offer suggestions on ways to make life easier. Excessive attention may be focused on day-to-day happenings and concerns unrelated to the disability, such as an argument with a friend or the extent of the student's involvement in extracurricular activities.

Students at our counseling center often supported the image of normalcy by expressing concern about a variety of "normal" symptoms, but they did not relate the disability to these other problems. For example, two diabetics were severely depressed and worried about "self-esteem," two students with cerebral palsy were contemplating suicide, one with lupus syndrome was worried about a relationship with a male, two postsurgical patients developed eating disorders, and one midget began with an interest in assertiveness training. (This may have been due, in part, to the student's belief that the counseling center dealt with psychological issues, not rehabilitation issues.) The disabled students frequently undertook many tasks that nondisabled students would not be expected to do and did them independently as if that were the norm.

Case Example: Enmeshment and Disengagement

Andrea, who had a moderate cerebral palsy, handled all the finances for her education, holding down a job for 20 hours a week on campus, obtaining and filling out financial aid forms, and working through the bureaucracy at the state rehabilitation agency to obtain educational benefits. Simultaneously, her parents showed overprotectiveness, and limited the distances and places they encouraged her to travel from home or campus, citing concern about financial or academic costs as the reason. They exhibited marked overinvolvement in their readiness to speak for Andrea, asserting that they knew what she was thinking, and questioned her in detail about her ups and downs of college living, such as disappointments with particular classes or roommates. Andrea invited such involvement with numerous complaints.

The rigidity of the boundary between Andrea and her parents, i.e., disengagement, is signified by the lack of mutual negotiation or exchange of information in the complex area of educational financing. Concurrently, a diffusiveness of the boundary, i.e., enmeshment, is revealed through the intensity and intrusiveness in issues Andrea could be expected to handle competently on her own.

Triadic Patterns of Conflict Management

In stressful situations, parents, children, and, frequently, grandparents may organize into triadic patterns for coping with conflict, such as triangulation, coalition formation, or detouring (Minuchin, 1974). Families with a disabled child may indicate that there are no problems in the family except for the complaints of the disabled child. Several couples treated at our center admitted to having contemplated divorce in the past, however, and one was divorced. Most of the children formed overt coalitions with the identified protective parent.

Case Example: Detouring

Paula was a diabetic who said she had been anorectic 6 months earlier. She was about 30 pounds overweight, had very high blood sugar readings, and played with her insulin dosages. Everyone agreed that Paula and her mother were very close. Mrs. S. was perceived as more worried about Paula's condition and more knowledgeable about it than Mr. S., who was less concerned about Paula's ability to regain control of her diet and insulin intake. Early in treatment, however, Mr. S. revealed that he had a heart condition as a result of his obesity. Whenever Mrs. S. would begin to confront Mr. S. with her worries about his health, he minimized her concern, and Paula turned the conversation to her own problems of "poor self-concept and low self-esteem."

When the wife begins to confront the husband, tension mounts. Paula's interception functioned as a distractor and diffused the parental conflict.

Adaptation to Change

The degree of rigidity or flexibility with which families respond to necessary change determines the extent of their efforts to maintain the status quo. Families with a handicapped member, like psychosomatic families, may maintain a rigidity in organization no matter what issues are discussed by the members. These families may be distinguished from families with psychosomatic concerns by their lifelong involvement with the problem. For families with a congenitally disabled child, activity may have been organized around detection of the disability, treatment, and care-giving since the child's birth. While the hopes and plans are theoretically intended to prepare this child for self-sufficient living, the organizational changes that allow the family to shift its focus from the disabled individual and provide greater autonomy for all the members have never been experienced by these families. The result is a reliance on the familiar and an inability to complete transactions intended to generate new outcomes. In our clinical sample, discussions about the child's autonomy after college often were aborted by an interactional reciprocity. It was almost as if the family myth was, "College is just a 4-year period of time to give you (me) a chance to feel normal, but you're (I'm) not normal, so we'll (I'll) endure until it's over and you (I) come home."

Case Example: Rigidity

Dan, a midget, was the only visibly disabled student on campus. He was being seen individually because his grades had declined dramatically and because he had accumulated numerous incompletes over 3 years. He had taken time off twice during his academic career, and now he was suggesting that he might do so again. He said his only option was to live at home, but he did not want to because his mother, a single parent, was too protective. During a family meeting with Dan and his mother to discuss the following academic year and the future, their inability to complete transactions was revealed. Whenever the therapist asked Dan's mother if she wanted Dan to finish college, she would respond either that Dan had probably done the best he could, that time was not important, or that it was better financially for him to be at home. Dan supported his mother by agreeing that this was not the time to finish, but said he would do it eventually. Neither Dan nor his mother responded with a definite "yes" or "no."

This lack of commitment to a response appeared to be the family's only available solution to the dilemma of whether the child should leave home. In a less rigid system, family members would perceive that choosing "yes" or "no" could lead to many possible actions.

Characteristic Pattern

In the structural model, these dimensions provide the data to hypothesize a response to the major assessment question: What function does this symptom serve in this family? While the general assumption on which the model is based is that the difficulties of the identified patient maintain family homeostasis, a specific pattern seemed to emerge for these families. In most, the father was identified as incompetent in some way and peripheral, and the mother was identified as competent and nurturing. The marital dyad was perceived to be in covert conflict by the therapist. One hypothesis is that the incompetence of the child stabilized the marriage by protecting the father from the mother's anger and unhappiness about his incompetent behavior.

CLINICAL CONSIDERATIONS

Family therapy with the disabled student in a college counseling center requires strategies that take into consideration the features inherent to the academic environment. Some conditions of this therapeutic setting are unique. For example, doubts have been raised about the prognosis for success of family therapy in a residential treatment setting (Haley, 1976). Although Haley was referring to mental health facilities, many of the reservations he expressed about residential placement also pertain to a college environment. Access to families is limited by the reality of geographical distance. In order to bridge this gap, it may be necessary to design tasks that link family members across the miles through telephone calls, strategic letters, or special visits. These strategies are not used exclusively in working with disabled students and their families.

Traditionally, it is presumed that college-aged adolescents should be developing independence and that the best way to do this is to experiment on their own. Like nondisabled students, disabled students often adamantly believe that their problem is exclusively theirs, and they refuse to have their family involved in finding a solution for fear of worrying family members unnecessarily. The therapist who requests the presence of the family in therapy may be perceived as someone who does not believe that disabled people can make it on their own. To gain maneuverability, the therapist may contract with a student for a limited number of sessions, usually six, in an attempt to resolve the problem. The therapist may suggest that, having conquered so many other problems, the student probably knows best how to handle this one, too. However (continues the therapist) it is possible that, out of concern for the family, the student may become confused about what to do. If the situation has improved in 6 weeks, the student was clearly right; if it has not improved, however, the reason must be that the student has realized the family should be included. This approach creates a therapeutic bind so that, whatever happens, the student is doing something positive.

In most mental health settings that provide family therapy, parents call with concerns about their child. In a college setting, more frequently either the child or the therapist calls to invite the parents into therapy. For the family of the disabled child, that telephone call can arouse their unspoken guilt feelings that they have not protected the child sufficiently and reawaken their worst fears that their child has failed at more independent living. Often, the disabled child states that one parent will come, usually the mother, but the other will never consent to participate in therapy. It is frequently helpful to call the peripheral parent; this avoids putting the overinvolved parent in the position of being turned down once more by the spouse already defined as "not caring." A simple introduction, followed by "I'm concerned about your son (daughter), and my guess is that you are, too. Would you and your wife (husband) come in and help me understand how best to help him (her)?" usually brings in the family. In such a message, the parents are presumed to be knowledgeable about the child's needs and influential in the child's life. Furthermore, it generally produces more relief than fear. When the family arrives, the therapist may have to reaffirm the expertise of the overinvolved parent, but the surprise at the cooperation of the more distant parent has already jolted the family organization enough to increase the maneuverability of the therapist.

Our college counseling center is neither a rehabilitation agency nor a medical facility; individuals and families tend to define the areas of expertise available there as psychological in nature. While there are staff members with varying levels of experience in rehabilitation at the center, resources from other services on campus are often used to ensure attention to needs other than sociopsychological needs. Disabled students who come to the center for help with psychological difficulties sometimes resent the intrusion of the therapist into the medical domain. This may make it difficult to deal with what the therapist views as the main problem (e.g., uncontrolled diabetes mediated by dysfunctional family transactions), especially if the family or individual insists that "poor self-esteem" or "depression" is the problem. Integrating the family's definition of the problem into the treatment plan can provide access to other aspects of the problem that need attention.

Case Example

> Matthew, a 20-year-old diabetic, called for an appointment at his mother's suggestion, because he was very depressed, could not find any reason to live, and wanted to drop out of college. Arriving with his mother, he appeared very sullen and complained about the college, his peers, his inability to stay physically fit, and just not "feeling good about himself." He was an avid runner (10 miles a day), but was eating very poorly. As an afterthought, he added that his blood sugar level was very high, and he was not following the physician's recommendations for insulin intake. When the therapist requested that Mr. W. be invited to the next session, Matthew said matters would only get worse with his father there. The therapist asked Matthew if he would help her by letting her know in the session when things were getting tense with his father present and asked Mrs. W. if it would be better if she or the therapist invited Mr. W. to come. Mrs. W. chose to ask him herself, and the next session included both parents.
>
> In fulfilling the eight-session contract, the therapist applied Haley's problem-solving therapy approach. The goals of the first family session were to decide whether Matthew should remain in school while solving his problems, to eliminate the threats or any real possibility of suicide, and to reduce the parents' sense of powerlessness in the face of these threats. Perhaps hoping that the therapist was more influential than they were, the parents decided that Matthew should stay in school. It became apparent that the parents were divided on many issues, including the explanation for Matthew's depression. Mr. W. thought the problem was poor self-esteem; Mrs. W. thought the problem was poor diet. Matthew

said "it" was his problem and nobody could help. When questioned, he said he probably was not going to commit suicide in the immediate future. To defuse the suicide issue, to reassure the parents, and to reinstate their sense of influence during the session, Matthew was told first to convince his parents that he planned to stay alive. Although the parents lived over 100 miles away, they were asked to alternate nights calling Matthew. Each was to advise him for only 3 minutes on his or her respective areas of concern. Since Mr. W. was also more convinced that Matthew would not attempt suicide, he was to spend 5 minutes a night reassuring his wife. The therapist asked Matthew to obtain the medical records and recommendations for the management of his diabetes from his physician. The therapist's goals were to make overt the covert cross-generational alliances of Matthew with each parent, to engage his father overtly in problem solving, and to begin to support the parents as the head of the hierarchy.

By the second session, the crisis mood had subsided, and the family was able to set behavioral goals to reflect the desired outcomes of "better self-esteem" and "improved diet." The therapist's goal was to unite the parents in helping Matthew behave in a productive and age-appropriate way. Several other problems emerged, including Mrs. W.'s great disappointment in Mr. W.'s management of his career.

A variation of the technique of developmental reframing (Coppersmith, 1981) provided the strategy for therapy. Briefly, the problem was redefined as one of age confusion. Matthew was chronologically 20, but sometimes acted as if he were 40, taking on his parents' problems. On the other hand, sometimes he behaved as if he were 12, becoming petulant, self-critical, and irresponsible about attending to his diabetic condition. The solution was to teach him to act his age. First during a session and then at home over vacation, when a behavior fit one of those age categories, the parents together held up an appropriate sign, labeled "12," "20," or "40," and gave an agreed upon response. The intent of this strategy was to help the parents take charge, to unite them in their responses to Matthew's behavior, and to strengthen the boundary around the parental subsystem. Matthew and his parents began to detect humor in the situation. His diabetes was under control by the end of therapy, he had gained a few pounds, he was more active with his peers, and he displayed a sense of humor. The parents seemed more optimistic about other family problems.

CONCLUSION

More and more frequently, disabled individuals and their families are using the process of going to college as a way to negotiate the leaving home stage of the family developmental life cycle. Although we have focused on college students, we believe that the concepts can be generalized to other treatment settings in which leaving home issues are being resolved. We also prefer to use the systems models of therapy at other transitional stages of family development, especially for the disabled, as these models of assessment and treatment transcend self-image, individual incompetence, and parental blame.

REFERENCES

Briard, F.K. (1976). Counseling parents of children with learning disabilities. *Social Casework, 57*, 581–585.

Coppersmith, E.I. (1981). A developmental reframing: He's not mad, he's not bad, he's just young. *Journal of Strategic and Systemic Therapies, 1*(1), 1–8.

DeLoach, C., & Greer, B. (1981). *Adjustment to severe disability: A metamorphosis*. New York: McGraw-Hill.

deParra, M.L.V. (1982). Changes in family structure after a renal transplant. *Family Process, 21*(2), 195–202.

Dunham, C.S. (1978). Role of the family. In R.M. Goldenson (Ed.), *Disability and rehabilitation handbook* (pp. 21–27). New York: McGraw-Hill.

Goldenson, R.M. (1978). Dimensions of the field. In R.M. Goldenson (Ed.), *Disability and rehabilitation handbook* (pp. 3–11). New York: McGraw-Hill.

Haley, J. (1973). *Uncommon therapy*. New York: W.W. Norton.

Haley, J. (1976). *Problem-solving therapy*. New York: Harper & Row.

Haley, J. (1980). *Leaving home*. New York: McGraw-Hill.

Jackson, D.D. (1967). The individual and the larger context. *Family Process, 6*(2), 139–155.

Minuchin, S. (1974). *Families and family therapy*. Cambridge, MA: Harvard University Press.

Minuchin, S., Rosman, B., & Baker, L. (1978). *Psychosomatic families*. Cambridge, MA: Harvard University Press.

Nigro, G. (1977). Sexuality in the handicapped: Some observations on human needs and attitudes. In J. Stubbins (Ed.), *Social and psychological aspects of disability* (pp. 131–136). Baltimore: University Park Press.

Peck, B.B. (1974). Physical medicine and family dynamics: The dialectics of rehabilitation. *Family Process, 13*(4), 469–479.

Ritterman, M.K. (1982). Hemophilia in context. *Family Process, 21*(4), 469–476.

Shapiro, R.J., & Harris, R.I. (1976). Family therapy in treatment of the deaf: A case report. *Family Process, 15*(1), 83–95.

Stanhope, L., & Bell, R. (1981). Parents and families. In J.M. Kauffman & D.P. Hallahan (Eds.), *Handbook of special education* (pp. 688–713). Englewood Cliffs, NJ: Prentice Hall.

Teismann, M.W., & Rodgers, B. (1982). A comparison of a traditional and a marital approach to rehabilitation counseling. *Journal of Marital and Family Therapy, 8*(2), 91–94.

Webb-Woodard, L., & Woodard, B. (1982). A case of the blind leading the "blind": Reframing a physical handicap as competence. *Family Process, 21*(3), 291–294.

Whiting, R. (1980). First semester freshmen college dropouts: A family system perspective. *Dissertation Abstracts International, 41A,* 951–952.

Wulfsberg, R.M. (1982). College enrollment patterns differ for handicapped students. *National Center for Education Statistics Bulletin* (NCES 80–B03). Washington, DC: National Center for Education Statistics.

4. Bearing the Burden Alone? Helping Divorced Mothers of Children with Developmental Disabilities

Lynn Wikler
Jane Haack
James Intagliata

You should know your chances of getting married again are lessened by having a handicapped child; you better face that in the beginning. (Divorced mother of a child with mental retardation)

W HEN SOCIAL CLASS IS HELD CONSTANT, NO SIGNIFICANT DIFFERENCE has been found between the divorce rate of parents of normal children and that of parents of children with developmental disabilities (Davis & MacKay, 1973; Roesel & Lawlis, 1983; Schufeit & Wurster, 1976). On the other hand, current estimates of divorce in the general population exceed one in every three couples (Ross & Sawhill, 1975). Given a 3% prevalence rate for mental retardation (PCMR, 1975), and that 20% of all children under 18 years of age reside in single parent homes, it can be estimated that 380,000 single parents are striving to raise a developmentally disabled child alone. While these families are headed by single fathers as well as single mothers, more than 90% of all children living with a divorced or separated parent live with their mothers (Bureau of the Census, 1981). Among developmentally disabled children living with a single parent, the proportion living with their mothers may be even higher.

The circumstances of those women who divorce and retain custody of their developmentally disabled child remain essentially unexplored (N. Robinson, personal communication, 1982). The results of extensive research and clinical exposition on the impact of a mentally retarded child on family functioning are available; nearly all, however, focuses on two-parent families (Gallagher, Beckman, & Cross). Although there is considerable literature on divorce and single parenting, most assumes normal cognitive development in the children. The compounded status of being a divorced mother and having a child with developmental disabilities has been neglected. Yet, these single parents are undoubtedly experiencing a great deal of distress.

It can be assumed from these combined literatures that the stressful circumstances facing the divorced mother of the child with developmental disabilities are greater than those facing either the divorced mother of a normally developing child or the married mother of a developmentally disabled child. Holroyd, Brown, Wikler, and Simmons (1976) indicated this to be true. When they analyzed stress levels reported by mothers, those in single-parent families reported significantly more stress than those in two-parent families. Similarly, Beckman (1983) found the only demographic variable significantly related to stress was the number of parents in the family; single parents reported more stress. She suggested that this finding was consistent with the main finding that increased care-giving demands were associated with higher levels of stress. "Single parents are likely to have less help with caregiving activities, since relief in the form of another parent is unavailable" (Beckman, 1983, p. 155).

Descriptive data on the family characteristics of institutionalized children indicate that single parents are more likely to place their mentally retarded children in an institution (Appell & Tisdall, 1968; Bayley, 1973; Graliker, Koch, & Hendersen, 1965; Hobbs, 1964; Saenger, 1960). Such trends in institutionalization could be explained by stress that is perceived as overwhelming and unending by the single parent. Given the current policy of supporting community-based care rather than institutionalization, these families would be seen as high risk for placement.

There is a possibility that the single-parent status of these women will be permanent. Single parents are often described as being in a transitional phase, i.e., they usually remarry within a few years of their divorce. Reported remarriage rates of divorced women range from 67% (Wattenberg & Reinhardt, 1979) to 80% (Glick, 1975), with 60% of remarriages involving children (Garfield, 1980). Factors that affect a woman's opportunity for remarriage include age, race, number of dependent children, and welfare recipiency (Ross & Sawhill, 1975; Wattenberg & Reinhardt, 1979). In exploratory interviews with single mothers of mentally retarded children, however, *none* of them stated any intentions to remarry, although several were in conjugal type relationships (Wikler, 1979). While some indicated that this decision was unrelated to the child who was mentally retarded, most acknowledged that the responsibilities of raising a chronically disabled child might preclude a partner from making a formal commitment. Therefore, the exacerbated stresses that these women experience in relation to their single-parent status may be long-term, and they may need appropriately long-term support services.

STRESSES OF DIVORCED MOTHERS OF CHILDREN WITH DEVELOPMENTAL DISABILITIES

Stresses of Child Care

The presence of children has been shown to be a central component of postdivorce distress (Berman & Turk, 1981). A single mother with custody is not a free social agent. Furthermore, she has the strain of meeting the practical and social responsibilities of raising a family. The ages of the children affect the way in which the mother handles this task; the burden of care is greatest if the children are very young and dependent (Hancock, 1980). Pressure on the divorced mother is intensified by the children's behavior (Hetherington, Cox, & Cox, 1976). Divorced mothers for whom income level is not a problem most often report stresses related to performing the maternal role alone, such as maintaining the house, caring for the children, and making arrangements for care during illness (Colletta, 1983).

The single mother of nondisabled children may be able to take time for herself because she has access to babysitters or can leave an older child unattended for brief periods during the day. In addition, her children may remain involved with their father, providing her some support in child care. It is more difficult for the single mother with a mentally retarded child to find substitute care (Cohen, 1982), and her children may have less contact with her ex-spouse (Wikler, 1979). In a survey of needs, single mothers with retarded children listed respite child care as their greatest need. They ranked financial needs second, and personal/social needs third. Single mothers with normal children listed these needs in the opposite order (Wikler, 1979).

The developmental disabilities of the child present special problems. First, the period of dependence is prolonged; it is as though the child is a preschooler forever. Second, the child may be hyperactive, have physical disabilities or unpredictable seizures, display inappropriate social behaviors, or communicate poorly. The extra care-giving demands, combined with the lack of social responsiveness in the child and temperament problems, are correlated with increased stress for the primary care-giver (Beckman, 1983).

The unrelieved responsibility of raising a chronically dependent person can drain the single mother's energy from such critical activities as developing new social relationships or managing a household routine. This strain, combined with the perception that it may never cease, places the single parent at increased risk for stress. The stresses that surround child care cannot be underestimated when working with the single parent of a mentally retarded child.

Financial Stresses

A major dilemma for any single parent is the strain of being both the primary care-giver and the primary wage earner. Women who head families and maintain independent households make up the largest proportion of the economically disadvantaged today (Norton, 1983; Wattenberg & Reinhardt, 1979). The Aid to Families with Dependent Children (AFDC) program is the primary source of income in 51% of these families, employment income for 28% of the families, Social Security payments for 12%, alimony or child support for 7%, and other income for 2% of the families (Wattenberg & Reinhardt, 1979). Several factors contribute to the poverty of these women. For example, they have the economic liability of being women; they earn approximately 57% of the income of the husband-wife family with the husband as wage earner (Bureau of Labor Statistics, 1978). In addition, they have shorter career ladders, less marketable skills, and less education, which lowers their potential earnings (Dinerman, 1977). A disproportionate number of single parents are nonwhite, which also reduces their potential earnings.

Colletta (1983) determined low income to be a key factor in the number of stresses reported by divorced women. Inadequate living arrangements related to downward mobility, unsatisfactory jobs, and the need to use welfare services were major issues. High levels of stress were, in turn, related to problematic child-rearing practices. Similar findings have also been reported in studying low-income single mothers. Intimate relationships were found to be helpful in mediating the impact of stress on parenting behavior, however. Federal and state financial subsidy programs have been available to help, but these programs are being cut by the current administration. For women with children under the age of 6 (generally the age group assumed to require a high level of care and supervision), it is probably more socially acceptable to receive AFDC or SSI benefits. As their children enter school, society expects these mothers to become economically self-sufficient.

There are additional reasons for financial difficulty for the single mother with a disabled child. First, the need for continuous child care and supervision generally does not end when the child reaches the age of 6; it may continue indefinitely. These mothers have fewer choices in pursuing full-time employment and may be too exhausted by child care demands to assume even part-time employment. Second, expenses are increased if the child has any special needs, such as specialized medical care that is not covered either by insurance or medical assistance, programming beyond the educational system, adaptive equipment, or extra child care costs.

Social Stresses

Social isolation has been strongly associated with divorce (Beck & Jones, 1970). Women mention their loneliness, isolation, and overwhelming responsibilities in almost every study of households headed by women (Wattenberg & Reinhardt, 1979). In a longitudinal study of single parents, Smith (1980) found them to be more isolated from their neighbors than their married counterparts. The absence of another adult within the household limits the availability of peer emotional support and assistance with various household tasks. Therefore, the single mother has less time and energy available for social activities and participation in community life.

The first 2 years of single parenthood are usually described as the most difficult, both socially and emotionally. At the same time that the mother must assume the increased child care or employment responsibilities for which she may not be fully equipped (Smith, 1980), she is also the loneliest. Relationships with relatives and friends are often disrupted. Gradually, a new friendship network forms with other women in a similar status, but until that happens, the mother is socially isolated—at a time when she most needs acceptance, intimacy, and respect.

Social isolation also characterizes two-parent families of mentally retarded children (Davis & MacKay, 1973; McAllister, Butler, & Lei, 1973). They are able to go out less frequently to visit friends, take vacations, or run errands together because of (1) maternal exhaustion from child care, (2) stigmatized social encounters, (3) special transportation needs, (4) the lack of babysitters or trained respite care providers at a reasonable cost, and (5) the loss of income that could be used for leisure activities as a result of the mother's inability to work outside the home. It is also often difficult to entertain at home, because of the minute-by-minute supervision needed by the retarded child, the amount of attention the child needs at night, and the child's inappropriate behaviors.

Given the increased levels of stress and social isolation reported both by single parents and by two-parent families with mentally retarded children, the mother with this *dual* status may be at even greater risk of stress. When the support networks of single mothers with a retarded child were compared with those of single mothers without a retarded child, it was found that almost one-third of the single mothers with a mentally retarded child were extremely isolated socially, with almost no supportive contacts through either formal or informal networks (Wikler, 1979).

Social isolation from peers and from the mainstream of the social environment has been correlated with child abuse and neglectful parenting (Bittner & Newberger, 1981; Marx & Newberger, 1982; Wayne, 1979). Parents who have no contact with other adults have limited access to support in times of trouble. Mothers who abuse their children are likely to report that they seldom see their relatives, feel that no one is interested in their problems, have experienced a death in the family recently, have little or no help with child care, disagree with their husband concerning discipline, have few relatives to count on, and see themselves as unconnected with others (Marx & Newberger, 1982).

Ironically, the personal dynamics that create a pattern of isolation can also maintain that isolation, frequently keeping such individuals from reaching out for or responding to overtures for help (Wayne, 1979). Services need to be geared toward the identification and aggressive support of single mothers of handicapped children who may be socially isolated.

Stresses of a Stigmatized Identity

Single parents of a child with mental retardation are likely to experience three types of social stigma that may interact to increase their social isolation and risk for emotional problems. The first stigma is the label *retarded*. The public's attitudes, in general, are governed by myths, stereotypes, and misconceptions regarding the label; these attitudes color people's interactions with those who are labelled mentally retarded (Dudley, 1983). The parents of children who are labelled mentally retarded may experience subtle avoidance, intrusive judgmental remarks, and even social ostracism. Although married parents also face this stigma, handling stigmatized encounters may be more difficult for the single parent.

Single mothers are also placed in another stigmatized role—that of being divorced. In a society with such a high divorce rate, people hold surprisingly negative attitudes about divorce, especially toward divorced women. Often, the single-parent family headed by a woman is referred to as a "broken" and "fatherless" family, while the two-parent family is referred to as "intact." Divorce is threatening in our couple-oriented society, as it challenges "family integrity." The recently divorced typically feel excluded, rejected, and alone. There is the added stigma in our success-oriented society of being a "failure" at marriage, making it even more difficult to admit one's loneliness (Woodward, Zabel, & Decosta, 1980).

Some of these women are placed in a third stigmatizing situation by being welfare recipients. There may be a financial crunch, often partly because child support payments are not forthcoming. Qualified full-time babysitters or day care providers who can meet the child's special needs and the burden of care are extremely difficult to find at a reasonable price. Without child care, the mother must stay at home, even if she prefers to work, and must utilize other sources of income. Regardless of her circumstances, however, dependence on taxpayers' money is frowned on in this society.

Emotional Stresses

Divorced people are overrepresented among psychiatric patients; they are more likely to develop physical illness, and they have higher morbidity rates than do comparable married people (Berman & Turk, 1981). They are heavy users of family services (Beck & Jones, 1970). The central component of the adjustment process is the individual's emotional reaction to the divorce itself and to life after the divorce. During the first postdivorce year, both men and women report low self-esteem, confusion regarding sexual values, and feelings of anger, anxiety, ambivalence, and depression. Women also report feeling unattractive, helpless, and personally and socially incompetent.

Following divorce, separation, or widowhood, the single mother must reintegrate her personal and emotional life by learning new skills and mastering loneliness. Major stresses include (1) pragmatic concerns, such as finances, home repair, maintenance; (2) emotional difficulties, such as the loss of the role as wife and the fantasy of "living happily ever after," loneliness, feelings of failure, and depression; (3) interpersonal problems, such as developing and maintaining friendships, as well as dealing with stereotypes and stigmatized attitudes; and (4) family-related problems, such as responding alone to the demands of raising children, finding enough time for the children, and dealing with the former spouse (Berman & Turk, 1981). The combined effect of all these stresses puts divorced mothers at risk for psychiatric problems.

Breakdown of a marriage after the birth of a mentally retarded child may be due to various marital problems, including the stresses of the all-encompassing child care, the mother's involvement with the child to the exclusion of the father, or problems in marital communication (Turner, 1980). The potential for overinvolvement with the mentally retarded child does not necessarily dissipate after divorce; in fact, it may increase without the counterbalancing effect of another adult presence.

The divorced woman may feel inadequate as a wife, and the mother of a disabled child may feel inadequate as a mother. Divorced women with disabled children thus have two losses to grieve, two areas of "breakdown" that they are helpless to repair. The children are tangible reminders of the marriage that ended, and the handicapping condition can exacerbate feelings of chronic sorrow (Olshansky, 1962; Wikler, Wasow, & Hatfield, 1981).

Stress of Lack of Information

Parents of mentally retarded children often complain that there is very little written on solutions to the day-to-day problems of raising a mentally retarded child (Matheny & Vernick, 1969). Most of this "tidbit" information must be obtained from other parents in the same situation (Weingold, 1968). Single mothers often complain that they do not know how to be a "father" *and* a mother to their child. Thus, single mothers with a mentally retarded child may have the combined frustration of not being sure how to father their child or how to mother their special child.

FAMILY INTERVENTIONS

Family Support Services

The most relevant initial clinical intervention is the provision of family support services. McLanahan, Wedemeyer, & Adelberg (1981) listed three components of support services to single parents:

1. direct services, such as respite care, information and advice relevant to the solution of specific problems, and in-home services to relieve the burden of care
2. emotional support, through relationships that provide security, intimacy, and reassurance of worth
3. social integration into community activities and access to new information and new social contacts

Family counselors who serve single mothers of disabled children should have knowledge of developmental disabilities, their implications for families, and available community resources. Case management and linkage skills are important in helping parents to utilize and coordinate available resources in the complex human services system (Intagliata, 1982). The family therapist not only should be able to act as an advocate to obtain and to create needed services, but also should be aware of community organization and social planning to effect change (Andrews & Wikler, 1981; Horejsi, 1979).

The family therapist must be sensitive to the mother's need for specialized information about the implications of the child's mental retardation now and in the future. At certain points, providing concrete information may be as beneficial to the mother as meeting her emotional needs. The emotional disintegration of the family following the divorce creates stress for the child. As the child grows older, other developmental and transitional points become stressor events with which the single mother must cope (O'Hara &

Chaiklin, 1980; Wikler, 1981a, 1983). Helping the mother anticipate and plan for these difficult periods can soften their impact.

Finally, the counselor should make a special effort to commend the single mother on her strength, her endurance, her activities, her energy, and her parenting creativity (Barry, 1983; Wikler, Wasow, & Hatfield, 1983). Without a spouse, she will be particularly appreciative of positive feedback for her parenting endeavors.

Family Network Therapy

A family therapist should assess the natural support network of the divorced mother of a child with a developmental disability. The presence of a severely mentally retarded child often alters interactions with extended family and community, as the family tends to disengage itself socially in order to focus on internal problems (Farber, 1968). These interactions are likely to change again during the first 2 years after separation and divorce. It is crucial for successful individual and parental functioning that a single mother be integrated into a viable psychosocial support system. This network can provide intimacy, maintain social identity, offer emotional support, and reduce daily stresses. The network should be suited to the mother's current situation.

The therapist should determine whether the family ties and old friendships have been maintained, reestablished, or disrupted; whether the mother believes her network is satisfying her needs; and whether the mother needs to meet new people who share her status and future orientation. An especially isolated single mother may need assistance in establishing a support network and relinquishing the privacy to which she has become accustomed. A single parent with a mentally retarded child may actually need a *stronger* support network than other people need.

If a single mother feels trapped or distressed, her support network may need attention. The support networks described by McLanahan and associates (1981) may prove useful as examples of how a single mother might develop or modify a support network. The type of structure and support provided is moderated by the availability of family and friends, and by the role orientation of the mother as a "stabilizer" (i.e., someone who tries to maintain predivorce roles) or as a "changer" (i.e., someone who attempts to establish a new identity). The networks are adaptive for different groups and may change over time. The support network discussed by McLanahan and associates (1981) includes

1. family of origin. The kinship ties with the mother's original family form one part of the support network. If they live nearby, family members are able to provide frequent primary support of direct services and emotional support. This does not ensure intimacy, however, and it decreases social integration by isolating the mother from community supports and new social experiences, making this type of network better for a stabilizer orientation.
2. extended network. Although the extended network consists primarily of new friendships, especially with other single mothers, it may include the ex-spouse, predivorce friends, and relatives. Men may be included, but they are not so important. There are usually large clusters of relationships, with different people providing different types of support (e.g., direct services, emotional support, social integration). There is a strong sense of shared commitment and experiences, with high social integration. This type of network is less stable because of the remarriage, mobility, and transience of its members. Some mothers with high levels of distress and a negative self-image may try to make their network more stable by continually expanding the number of its members.
3. conjugal networks. Some single mothers establish a conjugal family form by the presence of a spouse equivalent as the major source of support. Generally, the woman identifies with the wife/mother role. The first subtype includes old friends or relatives and is similar to the family-of-origin network in terms of benefits and risks. The second subtype is a conjugal relationship combined with a large and dense network (primarily of new friends), which is similar to the extended network. The latter subgroup of mothers are usually less dependent on the male bond and are more career-oriented. Often, single mothers move into one of these two conjugal networks from the extended network or family-of-origin network.

A functioning support network can be developed by broadening the definition of the client to include her social context. The family therapist can request meetings with the client and her parents, siblings, friends, and neighbors. The focus of such meetings varies according to the individualized needs of each client, but they should both reduce the single parent's social isolation by alerting her personal community to her needs and facilitate an active negotiation for exchange of services and emotional support among the participating members (Reuveni, 1979). This vision of the expanded role of a family therapist has been successfully realized with families of suicidal members (Reuveni, 1979), as well as with families of mentally retarded children (Berger & Foster, 1976; Slater & Wikler, 1983).

Family Therapy

The divorced mother of a child with developmental disabilities can often be helped by family therapy (Berger & Foster, 1981; Turnbull & Turnbull, 1982; Turner, 1980; Wikler, 1981c). There is substantial documentation of the acute distress experienced by each family member after a marriage has been dissolved (Wallerstein, 1983). There is also a clear interaction between the parent's level of functioning and that of the children during the postdivorce transition. A depressed and anxious mother is less adaptable, and her lack of emotional availability to the children can contribute to their intense, but usually temporary, dysfunction. In a 20-year longitudinal study, Chess, Thomas, Korn, Mittleman, and Cohen (1983) compared the adult adjustment of children of divorced parents with that of children of nondivorced parents and found no significant differences.

The psychological tasks of the postdivorce child are beautifully conceptualized by Wallerstein (1983), who described six issues that the child must resolve:

1. acknowledging the reality of the marital rupture
2. disengaging from parental conflict and distress and resuming customary pursuits
3. resolving the loss
4. resolving anger and self-blame
5. accepting the permanence of the divorce
6. achieving realistic hope regarding relationships

The child's ability to master these areas is critical and, in many ways, depends on the mother's process of regaining her morale.

Although the ways in which children with developmental disabilities adjust to divorce have not been explored, their responses are likely to be similar to those of nondisabled children, when matched for maturational age. In the past, mental health professionals have claimed that psychotherapy is not effective with mentally retarded children or adults. Current studies indicate the utility of such approaches, however (Hayes, 1976; Selan, 1976). Similarly, it is now recommended that the handicapped child be included in family therapy sessions relating to divorce adjustment (Turner, 1980).

Family therapy can accomplish several goals. First, relevant information can be shared with the family about the process of divorce and about the developmental disability of the child with less risk that the information will subsequently be distorted. Second, the family therapist can encourage open discussion among the family members. Families under stress often have neither the skills nor the inclination to share their emotions with one another. Avoidance of issues surrounded by tension can increase the isolation of family members, which reduces the family's ability to face the stresses. Third, the family therapist can observe and identify current family patterns that family members may not have recognized. By watching the family interact as a group, the family therapist can observe certain repeated dynamics and can intervene to promote a more constructive mode of interaction (Wikler, 1981c).

Mothers of children with developmental delays have often been clinically characterized as "overprotective." Behavioral coding of their interaction style indicates that mothers of handicapped children exhibit more maternal directiveness and less responsiveness to their child than do mothers of nonhandicapped children (Vietz & Anderson, 1981). Observations of families in treatment also showed enmeshment to be a clinical issue for the mother and disabled child (Ferrari, Matthews, & Barabas, 1983). The potential for this enmeshment is likely to increase when another adult is unavailable, i.e., in single-parent families. This overinvolvement could be problematic for several reasons; it may

- reduce the mother's opportunity to have her intimacy needs met through other adults, further isolating her
- increase the likelihood that the child will adopt the mother's dysfunctional approach to the handicap
- decrease the potential development of independence in the handicapped child
- interfere with appropriate development of the other children in the family

Structural family therapy has proved useful in disengaging the enmeshed dyad, enabling better ego differentiation, and clarifying boundaries. A family systems approach that included behavioral training has been shown effective in reducing the overinvolvement of the mother and reducing disruptive behavior of the child with developmental disabilities (Harris, 1982).

Group Therapy

Traditional counseling services for single parents and parents with mentally retarded children have focused more on individual assistance than on family therapy or group therapy. There is, however, a developing body of clinical literature on parent groups that have been formed to offer mutual aid and to share information. Relevant peers may be most capable of providing these parents with what they need (Loeb, 1977). In this case, those peers are other single parents with retarded children. Although there are organizations for single parents, such as Parents Without Partners, and for parents of mentally retarded children, such as the Association for Retarded Citizens, there is no organization focused on the combined status of being single and having a handicapped child. These parents may not find one another without a therapeutic structure.

Groups are an appropriate family treatment intervention not only because they reduce the single parent's social isolation, but also because they provide emotional support. In a group, these mothers can receive valued feedback from other adults who are experiencing similar stresses. This peer support can help reduce feelings of stress, "normalize" their life situation, and decrease their feelings of separateness. Peers can offer a new frame of reference in which each mother can contrast her own decisions with the experiences, responses, and expectations of others. After observing themes shared by several group members, these mothers are less likely to judge themselves so harshly; they can better validate their own accomplishments. By providing these women with a chance to talk about themselves and their stresses among peers, they can develop insight, strength, interpersonal skills, and a more accurate understanding of themselves and their situation.

A group leader can encourage single mothers with a mentally retarded child to establish a system for mutual aid so that each need not bear the burden of child care alone. A network of peers that can be called upon to exchange services is invaluable. This cooperative aid can involve help in practical areas, e.g., babysitting, cooking, transportation, housing, and sharing of material goods, as well as in emotional and information areas.

Groups can share specialized information on a disability and its implications over time. With a knowledge of other mothers' experiences, future planning may be easier. Sources of information generally unavailable to individuals, such as speakers or films, can be provided to groups because of the number of parents being served at one time. Behavior management techniques can be taught successfully in a parent group context (Rose, 1974). Skills such as advocating for the child's rights, negotiating a service delivery system, or dealing with stigma in a public setting can be developed in a group. Demonstrations and exposure to a variety of problem-solving situations help generalize learning and build confidence. The exchange of information, opinions, specific coping strategies, and suggestions can assist these mothers in dealing with day-to-day problems and can facilitate their problem-solving capabilities.

One group therapy approach that may be quite useful with single parents of developmentally disabled children was investigated by Intagliata and Doyle (1984), who trained a group of these parents in interpersonal problem-solving skills. Over the 3-month course of the training sessions, parents in the group realized two major benefits: (1) they were able to draw emotional support from each other by acknowledging and sharing their common stresses, and (2) they increased their competence in dealing with interpersonal problems and conflicts.

While the participants in the group could certainly apply the interpersonal problem-solving skills they learned to dealing more effectively with their disabled children, the training focused on ways that parents could use these skills to broaden and strengthen their social support networks. Assessment of the parents prior to the group training had, in fact, indicated that they were far more competent in dealing with child-related problems than they were in dealing with problems involving other adults (e.g., extended family members, co-workers, neighbors). As emphasized by Intagliata and Doyle (1984), good interpersonal problem-solving skills are especially important for parents of developmentally disabled children, since these skills may be essential in developing and maintaining the well-diversified base of social support that they need.

In sum, group work is an extremely useful, efficient, and effective family intervention for helping the divorced mother of a child with developmental disabilities. A parent can participate in a specialized parent group while receiving family support services, family network therapy, and family therapy. These various interventions are not incompatible, nor do they duplicate one another in their impact. Since long-term planning and support are advocated for these clients, these services could be offered sequentially and strategically over time.

REFERENCES

Andrews, S., & Wikler, L. (1981). Social work practice and developmental disabilities. *Health and Social Work* [Special Supplementary Issue], 625–685.

Appell, M.A., & Tisdall, W. (1968). Factors differentiating institutionalized from non-institutionalized referred retardates. *American Journal of Mental Deficiency, 73,* 424–432.

Barry, A. (1983). A research project on successful single-parent families. *American Journal of Family Therapy.*
Bayley, M. (1973). *Mental handicap and community care.* Boston: Routlege, Kegan, and Paul.
Beck, D.F., & Jones, M.A. (1970). Progress on family problems: A nationwide study of clients' and counselors' views on family agency services. In *Family Services Association Census Report,* New York: Family Services Association.
Beckman, P.J. (1983). Influence of selected child characteristics on stress in families of handicapped infants. *American Journal of Mental Deficiency, 88* (2), 150–156.
Berger, M., & Foster, M. (1978). Family-level interventions for retarded children: A multivariate approach to issues and strategies. *Multivariate Experimental Clinical Research, 2,* 1–21.
Berman, W.H., & Turk, D.C. (1981). Adaptation to divorce: Problems and coping strategies. *Journal of Marriage and the Family, 43* (1), 179–189.
Bittner, S., & Newberger, E.H. (1981). Pediatric understanding of child abuse and neglect. *Pediatrics in Review, 2* (7), 197–207.
Brandwein, R. (1977). After divorce: A focus on single parent families. *The Urban and Social Change Review, 10.*
Bureau of the Census. (1981). Marital status and living arrangements, March, 1981 (Series P-20, No. 372) Washington, DC: U.S. Department of Commerce.
Bureau of Labor Statistics (1978). *Marital and family characteristics of workers 1970-1978.* Washington, DC: U.S. Department of Labor.
Chess, S., Thomas, A., Korn, S., Mittelman, M., & Cohen, J. (1983). Early parental attitudes, divorce, and separation, and young adult outcome: Findings of a longitudinal study. *Journal of the American Academy of Child Psychiatry, 22* (1), 47–51.
Cohen, S. (1982). Supporting families through respite care. *Rehabilitation Literature, 43,* 1–2, 7–11.
Colletta, N.D. (1983). Stressful lives: The situation of divorced mothers and their children. *Journal of Divorce, 6*(3), 19–31.
Davis, M., & MacKay, D. (1973). Mentally subnormal children and their families. *Lancet,* October 27.
Dinerman, M. (1977). Catch 23: Woman, work and welfare. *Social Work, 22*(6), 472–477.
Dudley, J. (1983). *Living with stigma: The plight of the people who we label mentally retarded.* Springfield, IL: Charles C Thomas.
Farber, B. (1959). Family adaptations to severely mentally retarded on family integration. *Monographs of the Society for Research in Child Development,* (1, Serial No. 71).
Farber, B. (1968). *Mental retardation: Its social context and social consequences.* Boston: Houghton Mifflin.
Ferrari, M., Matthews, W., & Barabas, G. (1983). The family and the child with epilepsy. *Family Process, 22,* 53–59.
Garfield, R. (1980). The decision to remarry. *Journal of Divorce, 4*(1), 1–10.
Glick, P. (1975). A demographer looks at American families. *Journal of Marriage and the Family, 37*(1), 15–26.
Graliker, B., Koch, R., & Hendersen, M. (1965). A study of factors influencing placement of retarded children in a state residential institution. *American Journal of Mental Deficiency, 69,* 553–559.

Hancock, E. (1980). The dimensions of meaning and belonging in the process of divorce. *American Journal of Orthopsychiatry, 50*(1), 18–27.

Harris, S. (1982). A family systems approach to behavioral training with parents of autistic children. *Child and Family Behavior Therapy, 4*(1), 21–35.

Hayes, M. (1977). Psychotherapy with a mentally retarded child. *Smith College Studies in Social Work, 47,* 112–153.

Hetherington, E.M., Cox, M., & Cox, R. (1976, September). *The aftermath of divorce.* Paper presented at the meeting of the American Psychological Association, Washington, DC.

Hobbs, M.T. (1964). A comparison of institutionalized and noninstitutionalized mentally retarded. *American Journal of Mental Deficiency, 69,* 206–221.

Holroyd, J., Brown, N., Wikler, L., & Simmons, J.Q. (1976). Stress in families of institutionalized and noninstitutionalized autistic children. *Journal of Community Psychology,* 26–31.

Horejsi, C.R. (1979). Developmental disabilities: Opportunities for social workers. *Social Work, 24*(1), 40–43.

Intagliata, J. (1982). Improving the quality of community care for the chronically mentally disabled: The role of case management. *Schizophrenia Bulletin, 8,* 655–674.

Intagliata, J., & Doyle, N. (1984). Enhancing the social support networks of parents with developmentally disabled children: Training in interpersonal problem-solving skills. *Mental Retardation.* In press.

Loeb, R.C. (1977). Group therapy for parents of mentally retarded children. *Journal of Marriage and Family Counseling,* April, 77–83.

Marx, T., & Newberger, E. (1982, May). *Ecologic reformulation of pediatric social illness.* Paper presented at the annual meeting of the Society for Pediatric Research, Washington, DC.

Matheny, A.P., & Vernick, J. (1969). Emotionally overwhelmed or informationally deprived. *Journal of Pediatrics, 74*(6), 953–959.

McAllister, R., Butler, E., & Lei, T.L.J. (1973). Patterns of social interaction among families of behaviorally retarded children. *Journal of Marriage and the Family, 35,* 93–100.

McLanahan, S.S., Wedemeyer, N.V., & Adelberg, T. (1981). Network structure, social support, and psychological well-being in single-parent families. *Journal of Marriage and the Family, 43*(3), 601–612.

Norton, A. (1983, September). *Current demographics on the American family.* Paper presented at the National Institute of Child and Human Development Conference, Quail Roost, NC.

O'Hara, D.M., Chaikin, H., & Mosher, B.S. (1980). A family life cycle plan for delivering services to the developmentally disabled. *Child Welfare, 59*(2), 80–90.

Olshansky, S. (1962). Chronic sorrow: A response to having mentally defective children. *Social Casework, 43,* 190–192.

President's Committee on Mental Retardation (PCMR). (1975). *Mental retardation: The known and the unknown.* (DHEW Publication No. OHD 76-21008). Washington, DC.

Reuveni, U. (1979). The family therapist as a system interventionist. *International Journal of Family Therapy, 1*(1), 63–75.

Roesel, R., & Lawlis, G.F. (1983). Divorce in families of genetically handicapped/mentally retarded individuals. *American Journal of Family Therapy, 11*(1), 45–50.

Rose, S. (1974). Training parents in groups as behavior modifiers of their mentally retarded children. *Journal of Behavior Therapy and Experimental Psychiatry.*

Ross, H.L., & Sawhill, I.V. (1975). *Time of transition: The growth of families headed by women.* Washington, DC: Urban Institute.

Saenger, G. (1960). *Factors influencing the institutionalization of mentally retarded individuals in New York City.* Albany: NY State Interdepartmental Health Resources Board.

Schufeit, L.J., & Wurster, S. (1976). Frequency of divorce among parents of handicapped children. (ERIC Number ED 113-909). *Resources in Education, 11*(3), 71–78.

Selan, B.H. (1976). Psychotherapy with the developmentally disabled. *Health and Social Welfare 1*, February, 73–85.

Slater, M., & Wikler, L. (1983). *Normalized family resources: A new perspective on social support mobilization for families of children with developmental disabilities.* Working paper, Waisman Center, Madison, WI.

Smith, M.J. (1980). The social consequences of single parenthood: A longitudinal perspective. *Family Relations, 29,* 75–81.

Turnbull, H.R., & Turnbull, A.P. (1982). Parent involvement in the education of handicapped children: A critique. *Mental Retardation, 20*(3), 115–122.

Turner, A. (1980). Therapy with families of a mentally retarded child. *Journal of Marital and Family Therapy, 6*(2), 167–170.

Vietz & Anderson (1981). Style of parent-child interaction. In M. Begab, C. Haywood, & H. Garber (Eds.), *Psychosocial Influences in Retarded Performances.* Baltimore: University Park Press.

Wallerstein, J.S. (1983). Children of divorce: The psychological tasks of the child. *American Journal of Orthopsychiatry, 53*(2), 230–243.

Wattenberg, E., & Reinhardt, H. (1979). Female-headed families: Trends and implications. *Social Work, 24*(6), 460–466.

Wayne, J.L. (1979). A groupwork model to reach isolated mothers: Preventing child abuse. *Social Work with Groups, 2*(1), 7–18.

Weingold, J.T. (1968). Parents counseling other parents of retarded children. *Social Services for the Mentally Retarded and Their Families,* 575–580.

Wikler, L. (1979, June). *Single parents of mentally retarded children: A neglected population.* Paper presented at meeting of the American Association of Mental Deficiency, Miami.

Wikler, L. (1980). Folie a famille: A family therapist's perspective. *Family Process, 19,* 257–268.

Wikler, L. (1981a). Chronic stresses of families of mentally retarded children. *Family Relations, 30*(2), 281–288.

Wikler, L. (1981c). Family therapy with families of mentally retarded children. In A. Burman (Ed.), *Questions and answers in the practice of family therapy* (pp. 129–132). New York: Brunner/Mazel.

Wikler, L. (1983). *Periodic stresses in families of older children with mental retardation.* Paper presented at meeting of the American Association of Mental Deficiency, Houston, TX.

Wikler, L., Wasow, M., & Hatfield, E. (1981). Chronic sorrow revisited: Attitudes of parents and professionals about and adjustment to mental retardation. *American Journal of Orthopsychiatry, 5*(1), 63–70.

Wikler, L., Wasow, M. & Hatfield, E. (1983). Seeking strengths in families of developmentally disabled children. *Social Work,* in press.

Woodward, J.C., Zabel, J., & Decosta, C. (1980). Loneliness and divorce. *Journal of Divorce, 4*(1), 73–82.

5. Relationships of the Handicapped: Issues of Sexuality and Marriage

Gary L. Sanders

THE HANDICAPPED ARE USUALLY CONSIDERED BOTH PHYSICALLY AND mentally different from the nonhandicapped. They often suffer the added burden of social and sexual stigma. The difference between being handicapped and nonhandicapped does not need to be a negative one for sexual fulfillment, however.

Several authors have considered aspects of sexuality and marriage for the handicapped. For example, Peterson (1979) reviewed marital satisfaction in relation to role flexibility and role ambiguity. Nigro (1976) outlined her clinical observations of a diverse group of handicapped individuals and their intimate relationships. Sandowski (1976) examined clinical issues of paraplegia and sexuality. Munjack and Oziel (1980) covered the most significant biomedical aspects of disability and outlined methods of minimizing their impact. Bishop and Epstein (1980) presented a structured assessment and management schema for dealing with family problems and the disabled. Clearly, clinicians must deal with the marital and sexual problems of persons labeled handicapped.

DEFINITION OF HANDICAP

What constitutes an illness or handicap is defined by the sociocultural system in which it occurs. Poor eyesight is no longer considered a handicap in Western society, as methods of correction (eyeglasses) have been developed. However, the same eyesight would be a severe handicap in a more primitive culture in which people relied on hand-eye coordination and there was no means of correction. Thus, a handicap becomes such through the distinctions drawn by a particular society, group, or individual. Meyerson stated, "Society creates and exacerbates a handicap by identifying and labelling a 'condition' and by responding to or treating differentially persons so labelled" (cited in Peterson, 1979, p. 10). Almost any difference could be labeled a handicap at one time or another or in one culture or another. Our society emphasizes deficits in physical attraction and deficits in functional abilities as handicaps (Coet & Thornton, 1975).

THE IMPACT OF DISABILITY

Imagine a young woman who is wheelchair-bound because of polio. Her ability to move about is necessarily reduced. This one simple aspect of her disability can have a significant impact on the fulfillment of her life. Getting to a telephone takes so long that callers frequently hang up just as she approaches it. Getting to the door before the caller vanishes down the street becomes a major effort.

Imagine a 35-year-old married man, once the breadwinner of his family, respected by his community for his Little League coaching, now bedridden because of an industrial accident that crushed his spine at the neck. He has moved from independence to complete, exasperating dependency. He is treated like an infant and may even be spoken to like an infant.

Little imagination is needed to describe the impact of a disability on an individual. The impact is multiplied and complicated in the context of the couple. The young woman in the wheelchair has difficulty fulfilling her husband's expectations of her as a homemaker. The bedridden man no longer feels his wife's touch, and she notes he no longer takes interest in her sexually.

The impact of a disability on a couple can be enormous if one partner acquires a handicap after marriage. Both must adjust to changed self-images, to changed expectations, to physical limitations, and to physical differences. The development of their family may be altered because of lower fertility, decreased financial resources, or the concentrated effort required just to "make it" from day to day. The effects of a disability that was known before marriage can also affect the couple. This is obvious if the disability is progressive, such as multiple sclerosis, emphysema, or even arthritis. Even when the disability is static, such as missing limbs, neurological trauma, or postsurgical trauma, there is the opportunity for overprotection, infantilization, misunderstanding, stigmatization, and rigidity of social roles.

The sexual/marital problems and symptoms of the handicapped that may be brought to therapy are almost limitless. These concerns can appear separate from one another. For instance, a couple's concern over whether a spinal cord injury has altered fertility in the husband can be seen as predominantly sexual. If the same couple requests help in adjusting to the new marital role expectations, however, their concern can be seen as marital. These concerns can also appear quite entwined; for example, a wheelchair-bound wife's decreased sexual desire may be associated with the fact that valuable marital time together is now spent almost solely on solving the hassles of day-to-day living, leaving little or no time for emotional sharing.

BASIC ASSUMPTIONS

There are at least three basic assumptions that are useful to the therapist confronted with the marital or sexual concerns of the handicapped. A fundamental assumption is that presented symptoms can have multiple messages and multiple meanings. Their meanings may be in the realm of biologic understanding (e.g., pain signifying the reaching or exceeding of a physical limit), psychological understanding (e.g., pain signaling the perceived need to escape a threat), relationship understanding (e.g., pain as a message to the partner to draw closer and provide comfort), or systemic understanding (e.g., pain serving to bring the couple together or bring them to an outside helper). Since much of sexual functioning is directly dependent on biological functioning, a biologic understanding should be considered in sexual problems. By definition, marital problems are problems of relationship and require hypotheses of pattern and form. Sexual concerns can also be understood as secondary to process issues, however, and marital concerns as secondary to physical issues.

A second assumption is that not all problems require the same depth of treatment. That is, not all problems and symptoms need be nor should be dealt with by the same approach. Some problems may be best dealt with by direct advice, others by giving information, and still others by intensive therapeutic maneuvers.

The final assumption is that the goal of therapy is to provide an *opportunity* for the individuals within a given relationship to expand their options for personally perceived growth and personal satisfaction as they wish. It is important to defer to the couple's expertise in actually choosing their future path.

CLINICAL EVALUATION

Physical Evaluation

Many newly or progressively handicapped people see what is limited in their world, rather than what is not limited. It is, therefore, potentially useful for both the therapist and the couple to have *current* information on the handicapped individual's physical capabilities. A husband with a diabetic neuropathy that directly affects his erectile ability has a different choice of behaviors for future sexual activity than does a husband with no known organic causes for an erectile problem. Similarly, a wife with severe rheumatoid arthritis has different homemaking capabilities available to her than does the wife with little or no disability.

Coordination of Professionals

Depending on the specific nature of the disability, a number of different professionals may need to work together for the evaluation and treatment of the problem. For example, a wife who has lower limb paralysis secondary to polio and complains of sexual anesthesia needs a neurological evaluation for genital sensation and a pelvic examination by a gynecologist. When a handicap is progressive, it becomes even more necessary to involve various professionals in both evaluation and treatment. A spouse with progressive cancer needs repeated medical, physical, functional, and psychological evaluations to determine changing individual capabilities in addition to the ongoing interactional evaluations of marital or sexual therapy. This may well involve the combined efforts of the interactional therapist, psychologist or psychiatrist, internal medicine specialist, radiologist or immunotherapist, physiotherapist, occupational therapist, and the family physician.

The information obtained during evaluation is most useful for the marital subsystem; the therapist acts merely as a translator of the data. It is the couple who must eventually choose what alternatives to their interactional symptoms they want to try.

Evaluation of the Symptoms' Message

A component of evaluation relates to assessing symptoms as interactional messages. In evaluating the potential message behind the symptoms, the clinician should start with a simple understanding and move toward a more complex explanation only if necessary. This permits the clinician to deal with the couple's concerns by using the most appropriate and most economical resources.

Sexual concerns can more often be effectively understood and dealt with through more simple constructs than marital concerns. Relevant information and examples of sexual relationships are less available than demonstrations of marital relationships. For instance, depression in a handicapped husband who is unable to attain useful erections may be a "request" for permission to be different from how he was before or how he expects to be; on the other hand, the symptom of depression may be seen as a request by the couple for permission from the "authoritative" clinician to be different as a couple.

Symptoms may mean simply a lack of information. Long-term disabilities, particularly lifelong disabilities, may amount to a form of sociocultural deprivation that precludes the handicapped person from acquiring the social skills necessary for developing intimate relationships and problem-solving capabilities necessary for resolving difficulties.

The symptoms may also be seen as outlining a perceived lack of opportunities as a result of changes secondary to the disability. Peterson (1979) used the concept of disability time to describe the physically handicapped individual's time frame. The handicapped individuals described by Peterson frequently commented on the often significantly longer time required to perform everyday tasks. Need fulfillment from shared marital and sexual opportunities may take more time for the handicapped spouse. The nondisabled spouse must develop patience and slow the pace of each activity, as well as create longer spaces between activities.

The symptom cannot always be sufficiently understood through more simple message constructs based on physical functioning and its direct effects. This is particularly true of many marital concerns. In these cases, the symptom may be most usefully hypothesized as a systemic metaphor. The therapist hypothesizes as to the symptom's possible interactional *adaptive* function for the couple's relationship, determining the closeness of fit of the hypothesis through thoughtful questioning of the couple.

INTERVENTION: PLISSIT

Having evaluated, with referred help if necessary, the marital pair's priority problems, the clinician must determine the most appropriate level of intervention. It is important to remember that any interaction with the couple is a form of intervention, the effects of which must be assessed. There is no formula for predicting with certainty the best strategy in a particular case. The PLISSIT model of Annon (1974) helps the clinician to organize a hierarchy of interventions, however. PLISSIT is an acronym for Permission, Limited Information, Specific Suggestion, and Intensive Therapy.

Case Example

> Jack and Susan B. asked the therapist to help them regain what they called a normal marital and sexual life. Jack, 46, and Susan, 45, had been married 20 years and had chosen not to have children. It had been discovered 3 years ago that Susan was suffering from multiple sclerosis. Ever since the diagnosis, the couple's sexual contact had been decreasing to the point that there was virtually none at the time they sought therapy. Susan said this was because she had intermittent genital anesthesia or, on other occasions, hyperesthesia (excessive feeling, often to

the point of pain). She said that, because of this, she found intercourse uncomfortable and unpleasant. Jack, on the other hand, thought that Susan was simply avoiding sexual activity and asked the therapist if Susan could be going through menopause. He had noticed for the last 3 or 4 years that Susan's moods were very changeable. Susan denied that she was menopausal, said that her periods were regular, and added that the women in her family did not usually go through menopause until their late 40s. The lack of sexual contact had strained the rest of their marriage so that they seldom spent time together, other than at their unsatisfactorily prepared meals. Both identified their sexual life as the most disturbed aspect of their marriage.

Permission

A couple may simply require permission from an "authoritative" source either to continue as they have been or to make certain changes. Permission is used only in the context of the couple's specific concern, however. For example, the couple may simply require permission to try different sexual behaviors, to use fantasy, or to change their marital roles. Blanket permission is not useful.

The therapist may begin the intervention with Jack and Susan, for example, by giving them permission not to have genitally focused sex because of Susan's symptoms. They may be given permission to have other forms of physical contact, which each may have desperately wanted, but was afraid would ultimately lead to the current unpleasantness of intercourse. Perhaps most importantly, the therapist may give Jack and Susan permission to be true to their own sexual interests and desires so as not to enslave themselves to what each thought was the other's best interest. Such permission from the therapist may be all that some couples need. Jack and Susan may be set free by the permission so that they can creatively experiment with sexual activities other than just intercourse. If this permission is not sufficient, however, the next level of intervention is needed.

Limited Information

In dealing with issues of perceived difference (e.g., disability or sexual dysfunction), the dissemination of limited information is frequently all that is required. The information given should address the couple's priority concerns. It may cover specific physical information, perhaps anatomy, physiology, normal sexual development, conception, contraception, or effective sexual stimulation. It may also include nonphysical information related to the prevailing societal attitudes and behaviors toward disability and sexual activities, the myths and ignorance surrounding sex and handicapped people, or the nature and effect of sexual and marital role typing. Information can be provided in a number of different means, such as direct discussion, bibliotherapy, audiovisual aids, or referral to a preferred specialist. Limited information is most often used in connection with some form of permission.

It may be useful, for example, to tell Jack and Susan about multiple sclerosis in more detail. They may find it helpful to know that recurrent exacerbations of the symptoms with relative symptom-free periods are common and that many women with multiple sclerosis also suffer unpredictable changes of mood. The couple could be informed that many couples with similar problems discover forms of sensual and sexual exchange that do not depend on intercourse, yet still meet their needs for intimacy. Perhaps, for Jack and Susan, the lack of information kept them focused on unsuccessful solutions. Giving them information specific to their problems may allow them to find more creatively useful solutions.

Specific Suggestions

The therapist may prescribe specific behaviors or patterns of behavior in a direct attempt to help a couple. Therefore, the clinician must determine what types of problem solutions the couple has already attempted. The suggestions address the couple's concerns directly and are described in detail. The clinician may prescribe such things as physical sharing without intercourse, advise the nondisabled partner to operate on disability time when with the disabled mate, or recommend marital time-outs in which one spouse decides on an outing for self-pleasure and the other spouse acts as the obligatory companion in order to observe the pleasure of the first. Follow-up is necessary to assess the usefulness of the suggestions.

If the combination of permission and limited information is not successful for Jack and Susan, specific suggestions may be employed. A more detailed behavioral history is needed for this approach (Munjack & Oziel, 1980). Specific suggestions may include a recommendation that both read some lay-oriented literature on multiple sclerosis and perhaps contact the local MS Society. These actions may provide not only further information on the nature and effects of multiple sclerosis, but also a potential forum for discussion of personal concerns.

More specifically, the clinician may prescribe sensual touching sessions designed to provide successive successes in a nonperformance context. Intercourse could be banned for the "time being" in order to avoid practicing "more of the same" unsuccessful habits. Describing the prescribed activities and responses in personal diaries can also be recommended. Banning intercourse, yet prescribing sensual exchange, may help to recontextualize physical sharing as nondemand and enjoyable for itself. Marital time-outs may help Jack and Susan rediscover why they were attracted to each other originally.

If follow-up shows that these types of specific suggestions are not useful to Jack and Susan or if the therapist notices "resistance" (i.e., failure to complete tasks or sabotage of tasks), intensive therapy is indicated.

Intensive Therapy

When the first three interventions have not enabled the couple to create a nonsymptomatic solution to their concerns or when the clinician determines that the couple requires more than purely directive intervention, the more in-depth family, marital, and sexual therapies are used. The clinician must have interpersonal process-oriented therapeutic skills and the agreement of the couple for therapy.

The Milan therapy notions of hypothesizing, neutrality, and circularity (Selvini Palazzoli, Boscolo, Cecchin, & Prata 1980) may be used. For example, the therapist in the case of Jack and Susan may hypothesize that the desire discrepancy with its subsequent marital arguments and counterblame is a functional attempt to maintain marital closeness (although attended by discomfort) without having to confront the full impact of the ongoing illness. After discovering from the information given by the couple that this hypothesis explains the pattern of their relationship equally as well, but more completely, than do their own ideas (i.e., she is sick, he is uncaring), the therapist can devise a systemic intervention. This may take the form of a systemic opinion (e.g., positively connoting the couple's adaptive solution and cautioning them against major or rapid change) or a prescribed ritual (e.g., alternating days of "pretending" to be married as they would want with days of "pretending" to be unmarried). These types of interventions are aimed at deeper levels of connectedness in the couple's overall relationship. In addition to introducing the unexpected, the opinion and ritual could challenge the deeper belief that there is only one correct way of understanding the symptoms. The discovery that there are equally valid and experientially connected alternative realities opens the door for finding one that meets the same functional needs without the same symptoms.

The reader is referred elsewhere (Selvini Palazzoli, Boscolo, Cecchin, Prata, 1980; Tomm, 1982) for a more comprehensive discussion. Other more directive approaches have also been described (Bishop & Epstein, 1980).

Clinical Case Example

The following case example illustrates the highlights of this discussion.

Lynn, a 33-year-old homemaker, and Ed, a 38-year-old chartered accountant, were referred by a neurologist because of Ed's difficulty in maintaining an erection sufficient for intercourse and intravaginal ejaculation. Married for 12 years, the couple had an 8-year-old son and a 3-year-old daughter. They had moved across the country 1½ years earlier because of a promotional transfer within Ed's company.

The problem had begun approximately 4 years before they sought therapy and had become worse since their move. The couple reported a satisfactory sexual life before the onset. Each was willing to initiate sexual contact, and each had the option of a full sexual response cycle during sexual activity. Ed's inability to "complete," as Lynn stated, sexual activity over the previous 4 years had caused much turmoil and dissatisfaction for both, but more so for her.

Ed had a 6-year history of intermittent spastic paresis of the lower limbs, with a 4-year history of permanent right toe drag and marked decreased sensitivity in his lower limbs. Since the move, in an effort to prove himself in a new workplace, Ed had spent much time away from home. Lynn's social support system was based across the country, and she felt trapped and alone. Because of his illness and his fear that he might not be able to support the family in the future, Ed had begun to encourage Lynn to become more independent. She, however, interpreted this to mean that he was trying to push her out of her homemaker's role.

The couple had attempted oral genital contact to relieve Lynn of sexual tension; this had been modestly successful. They had also attempted morning intercourse when Ed's reflex erections were strongest. This had been unsatisfactory. Avoidance had become their major method of dealing with their concerns.

Treatment was organized along four phases. The first phase consisted of a more thorough physical evaluation. Ed was asked to see his neurologist for a complete assessment and to have his records sent to the therapist. His progressive sensorimotor disability was outlined by the neurologist; Ed's markedly decreased physiological capability for erection was the result of spinal cord degeneration. This information was discussed at length with the couple.

In the second phase of treatment, the couple was given information, through slide-tape demonstrations, and frank discussions with the therapist, regarding normal sexual functioning and the alternatives available for sexual satisfaction that were not dependent on erectile capability. They were not told to act on any of this information, however. The couple was also given "permission" to be symptomatic and mutually unhappy at this stage. They were told that, because they had been through a great deal of stress as a result of moves and uncertainty about the illness, it was to be expected that they would have symptoms as a couple. Later in therapy, they were given permission to be creative.

The therapist precribed specific tasks during the third phase, such as sensate focus (nongenital initially and later including genitals if so wished), couple time-outs, bibliotherapy, and self-exploration exercises. The fourth phase involved "handing" therapy over to the couple. Ed and Lynn were put in charge of their own task generation and used the therapist only as a consultant. In all, including follow-up, there were 10 sessions. Throughout most of therapy, Lynn appeared less creative and more hurried than Ed. Lynn would also state that a return to intercourse was more important to her than to Ed.

Therapy was never formally ended, but left open to the discretion of the couple in the future. At the 3-month follow-up, intercourse had not occurred because of Ed's inability to maintain an erection. The couple had continued some of the tasks prescribed earlier, particularly sensual touching and time-outs. They agreed that intercourse was no longer needed, as they were able to attain erotic stimulation through touch sensation. Lynn had become more creative, both sexually and maritally, and was able to enjoy sensual and sexual activities that she had in the past considered only a precursor to intercourse or somehow "not nice." In addition, Lynn showed more flexibility in her homemaker role, pursuing some of her own special interests. Both described their marriage as more rewarding and fulfilling. In fact, Ed said to the therapist, "I wish we had discovered the sensuous pleasure of being lost in touch when first married—we may have given up intercourse then."

CONCLUSION

The therapist, whether with intent or not, acts as a constructivist with patients through the drawing of certain distinctions about the relationship and the environment (von Glasserfield, 1983). This is most obvious when applying certain labels such as disabled/nondisabled, handicapped/nonhandicapped, ill/well, and so on. It is equally important, however, in less obvious cases, such as when the therapist hypothesizes and inquires about the patterns and form of the relationship.

The goal of therapeutic intervention with handicapped couples displaying symptoms of marital and/or sexual dysfunction becomes one of increasing the couple's effective opportunities for choice between alternative distinctions (Keeney, 1983). This may best be accomplished through relying on the assumptions that symptoms are messages with multiple meanings; problems are best treated differentially, starting with the most simple and direct methods; and patients should be supported in "creating" their own future "reality," as opposed to having to accept the therapist-specified reality.

REFERENCES

Annon, J.S. (1974). *The behavioral treatment of sexual problems* (Vol. 1). Honolulu: Honolulu Enabling Systems.

Bishop, D.S., & Epstein, N.B. (1980). Family problems and disability. In D.S. Bishop (Ed.), *Behavioral problems and the disabled: Assessment and management*. Baltimore: Williams & Wilkins.

Coet, L.J., & Thornton, L.W. (1975). Age and sex: Factors in defining the term "handicap." *Psychology Reports 37*(1): 103–106.

Keeney, B. (1983, June). *Cybernetics of therapeutic change*. Paper presented at the Second Annual Conference of the Canadian Association for the Treatment and Study of Families (CATSF), Ste. Marguerite.

Munjack, D.J., & Oziel, L.J. (1980). *Sexual medicine and counseling in office practice*. Boston: Little, Brown.

Nigro, G. (1976). Some observations on personal relationships and sexual relationships among lifelong disabled Americans. *Rehabilitation Literature, 37*(11/12), 328–334.

Peterson, Y. (1979). *Marital adjustment in couples of which one spouse is physically handicapped*. Palo Alto, CA: R.E. Research Associates.

Sandowski, C.L. (1976). Sexuality and the paraplegic. *Rehabilitation Literature, 37*(11/12), 322–327.

Selvini Palazzoli, M., Boscolo, L., Cecchin, G., & Prata, J. (1980). Hypothesizing, circularity, neutrality: Three guidelines for the conductor of the session. *Family Process, 19*(1), 3–12.

Tomm, K. (1982). The Milan approach to family therapy: A tentative report. In D.S. Freeman & B. Trute (Eds.), *Treating families with special needs*. Ottawa: Canadian Association of Social Workers.

von Glasserfield, E. (1983, July). *The Process of Reality Construction*. Paper presented at the Sixth Biennial Mental Research Conference, San Francisco.

6. The Elderly and Their Families: An Interactional View

Wendy L. Watson
Lorraine M. Wright

What is the perfect picture of aging? Old King Cole being merry? Ol' man river just rollin' along? An old owl and old man of the mountain exuding wisdom? Society's view of aging is often that of deterioration, depression, dependency, dereliction, and, of course, death. In his crusade against this agist portrait, Comfort (1976) educated the "now" and the "new" old about the facts and falsehoods of aging by presenting the aged as achievers. Pointing out the political, artistic, anthropological, and philosophical feats of individuals in their later years, Comfort reveled in the profiles of persons such as Golda Meir, Ghandi, George Bernard Shaw, Margaret Mead, and Bertrand Russell. Comfort's 8 by 10 inch glossy of "old age as triumphant" is initially appealing; like the agist image of "old age as tragic," however, it promotes a homogeneous view of the elderly. The greatest handicap of the elderly may be the assumption that all are alike or the belief that age is a handicap. Rather than age itself, the response of the aged and their families to the older person's mental and physical health symptoms may be the handicap.

Generally speaking, there is a positive correlation between advancing age and the incidence of physical and psychological problems. According to Brody and Kleban (1983), the elderly experience an average of four symptoms daily. They found that pain and fatigue/weakness were bothersome to three-fourths and two-thirds of their elderly respondents, respectively. Of their elderly subjects, 55% experienced mental health problems, such as depression, anxiety, sleep difficulties, loneliness, and boredom on a day-to-day basis, while 52% experienced daily worries about their family, friends, and themselves (i.e., their cognitive decline, physical health, and ability to perform daily tasks). Upsetting events were troublesome to 43% of the elderly, while 20% to 30% of the elderly were bothered by nocturia, digestive discomfort, and colds/fever.

PHYSIOLOGICAL PROBLEMS OF AGING

Among the most common physiological changes associated with aging are

- an increase in high-frequency deafness, especially in males
- a decrease in visual acuity, particularly night vision
- a decrease in the amount and depth of sleep
- an increase in the duration of a response to a stimulus, which contributes to a decreased ability to do two things at once

- an increased sensitivity to drugs
- a decreased ability to distinguish blues from greens
- an increased sensitivity to glare
- a decreased flexibility of joints
- an increase in the occurrence of chronic conditions, such as heart disease, hypertension, arthritis, diabetes, and stroke

Signs and symptoms of physical illness may be absent or diminished in the elderly. For example, because of changes in nerve sensitivities, the aging patient may not experience the classic chest pain of younger associates during a heart attack. The aging patient may not develop a fever in response to infection because of a decreased ability to generate white blood cells. These differences in the manner in which physical ailments may appear makes it necessary to approach a diagnosis of hypochondriasis in the elderly with much caution. The complaints of an aged person, such as "Something isn't quite right. I just don't feel like myself today," should not be casually disregarded.

Physical disease in the elderly may manifest itself as a change in thinking. Confused thinking, produced by an insufficient supply of blood to the brain, may be the only symptom of the onset of a heart attack in an elderly person. The adult child's diagnosis of a parent's condition may be senility, while the pneumonia that is causing inadequate oxygen flow remains unidentified. Before considering the interactional and psychological aspects of confused thinking, the prudent family therapist investigates possible physical origins, recommending a thorough physical examination in search of something reversible and treatable.

A change in thinking may indicate acute brain syndrome induced by drug toxicity, heart attack, infection, stroke, or dehydration. It may also indicate chronic brain syndrome caused by Alzheimer's disease in 75% of cases. Generalized loss of intellectual functions with a slow and uncertain onset characterizes chronic brain syndrome. The elderly person with this syndrome may experience difficulty making decisions, understanding conversations, and recalling recent events. Finally, there is a loss of remote memory.

In the initial stages of chronic brain syndrome, the person's appropriate social behavior masks the intellectual decline, but suspiciousness, moodiness, and bizarre tales may follow. The elderly person is usually aware of these changes and becomes depressed. In the latter stages, however, the person is unaware of these thinking difficulties.

Herr and Weakland (1979) cautioned those working with families of the aged to avoid the assumption that a decline in mental functioning is a part of normal aging or "hardening of the arteries." The influence of maladaptive interaction should be considered before the dreaded label *senility*, which most professionals designate as a wastebasket term, is imposed on the elderly person with the concomitant hopelessness and lack of treatment.

PSYCHOLOGICAL PROBLEMS OF AGING

The impact of aging on an individual is difficult to predict because of the interplay between physiological and psychological functioning, as well as the eminent influence of context. Factors such as the amount of change experienced at one time, the pace of the change, the supports available, and the individual's history of coping with change all affect the aging adjustment. The systems concept that a change in one part affects every other part seems to be particularly salient in the life of the aging person. One physiological change increases the person's susceptibility to other physiological changes and may induce psychological and sociological changes in the aged person's world. Psychological and sociological changes can, in turn, affect the elderly person's physical health.

Multiple losses, such as loss of work, independence, mobility, home, spouse, friends, and income, impinge on the elderly person's sense of well-being, contributing to loneliness and depression. Loneliness is one of the most common problems of aging parents, according to the information garnered by Hirschfield and Dennis (1979) from 100 unstructured interviews with the children of aging parents, gerontological professionals, and aging parents themselves. Depression has been identified as the most widespread psychological problem among the elderly (Kaplan, 1979).

PROBLEMS OF AGING AND THE FAMILY

Robinson and Thurnher (1979) found that an adult child's perception of an elderly parent's independence and success with aging was a "source of comfort and reassurance to the child" (p. 590) and contributed to a positive intergenerational relationship. Conversely, the morale of the adult child and, subsequently, the affective quality of the elderly parent-adult child relationship were found to be diminished when the predominant interaction was based on the care of the elderly parent (Robinson & Thurnher, 1979).

Studying a similar context of elderly parent-adult child interaction, Zarit, Reever, and Bach-Peterson (1980) measured the level of burden experienced by the primary care-givers of impaired elderly. These burdens were described as "lack of time for oneself, the excessive dependency of the patient on the caregiver, and [the] caregiver's fears about further deterioration in the patient's behaviour" (p. 652). The results of this investigation indicated that the level of burden experienced by the care-giver was not related to the behavior problems caused by the impairment of the elderly person, but was associated with the social support the care-giver received (specifically, the number of visits of other family members to the elderly parent). This association was a negative correlation; the greater the perceived support system, as indicated by the number of visits, the lower the level of burden experienced by the care-giver.

When Lieberman (1978) asked 1,100 Chicago adults about the significant changes in their lives during the past 4 years, a change in a parent or parent-in-law was the second most frequently reported change, exceeded only by the death of a significant other. Of the total sample, over 50% of those with living parents had perceived a major change in a parent, and 40% of those found this parental change very troublesome to them personally. Adult children reported a deterioration in the parent's health or a parent's increased need for moral support three times more frequently than they reported a problem with a parent's finances. The impact of a change in the parent on the adult child was not related to the physical or psychological distance between the parent and the adult child.

In a seminal study of adult children and their view of problems with aging parents, Simos (1973) found that the children could cope with the physical problems of their parents, even though they required considerable time and attention. The psychological problems, the interpersonal problems, and the social problems of isolation or ineptness of their elderly parents was more disturbing. The children responded to their perception of these problems by

> attempting to console or comfort the parent, struggling with negative feelings aroused by the parent, serving as peacemaker with caretaking personnel and others, dealing with family disruptions sets off by the parent, or in rare cases attempting to limit the parent's insatiable demands. (p. 80)

Silverstone and Hyman (1976) indicated that children of aging parents respond with feelings of guilt, helplessness, and resentment when they perceive loneliness, depression, and dissatisfaction in their elderly parents.

INTERACTIONAL ASPECTS OF AGING

An examination of the cybernetic aspects of family interactions can reveal vital information about the elderly, their problems and potentials, and the impact of aging on the family.

- What is the cycle of family interaction that maintains or escalates the problems of the elderly?
- What continues to create concerns and complications for other members of the aging person's family?
- What behaviors, thoughts, and feelings of each family member perpetuate the maladaptive interaction?

Kramer and Kramer (1976) indicated that vicious cycles "accelerate like a spinning gyroscope and that gyroscopic effect is more powerful than the simple sum of the two [original behaviors]" (pp. 36–37). Circular pattern diagrams (Tomm, 1980) can be utilized to clarify the vicious cycles in which the family of an elderly person may be trapped. The cognition, affect, and behavior of each family member can be diagrammed.

Case Example: Depression

A middle-aged daughter observes her 72-year-old mother reminiscing and weeping. The daughter interprets this to mean that her mother is not happy now, inferring that she, as a daughter, has not been fulfilling her filial responsibilities. She feels guilty and attempts to cheer her mother by changing the topic. Her mother interprets this to mean that her daughter is not interested in her. The mother feels sad (initially, she had felt nostalgic), cries, and wishes for days past. The daughter observes this crying, and the cycle begins again, culminating in depression for the elderly parent (Figure 6–1).

Case Example: Confusion/"Senility"

A dutiful daughter visits her aged mother only to find the stove left on and her mother unable to tell her when she turned it on. Her mother cannot locate her glasses and becomes so overwhelmed in the face of her daughter's questioning that she cries. The daughter perceives these behaviors of her mother's as "senile." (Behavior that is termed "forgetful" in a 20-year-old and "preoccupied" in a 50-year-old is quickly labelled "senile" in an 80-year-old). The daughter is worried and feels

Figure 6–1 Vicious Cycle: Depression

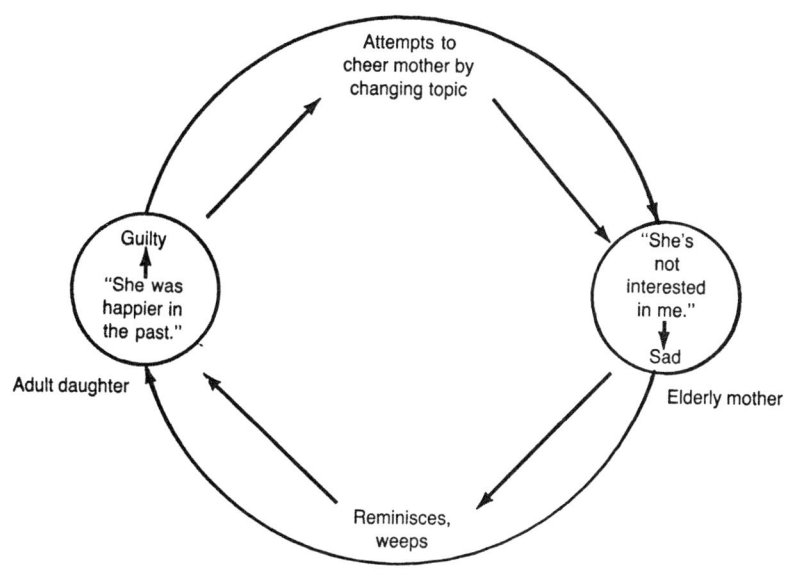

she should observe and take care of her mother for a while. She decides, without consulting her mother, that the best solution is for her mother to live at her (the daughter's) home. She neglects to orient her mother to the new living arrangements and to the daily routines, however, becoming impatient and abrupt with her mother's questions. Perceiving this impatience and quick change of scenery, her mother deduces, "I'm a burden. I'm so confused." Her anxiety about being an encumbrance and her fear about not thinking clearly further block her normal functioning, and the cycle escalates (Figure 6–2).

Case Example: Hypochondriasis

An elderly father talks of his physical pain and discomfort to his son, who feels frustrated and impotent, not knowing what to do. The son responds by trying to distract his father or by not commenting at all. The father interprets this behavior to indicate that his son just does not understand the seriousness of his condition or does not believe him. He feels rejected and worried, which drives him to talk more explicitly about his symptoms, e.g., "The pain is right over here, and it hurts when I get up

Figure 6–2 Vicious Cycle: Confusion

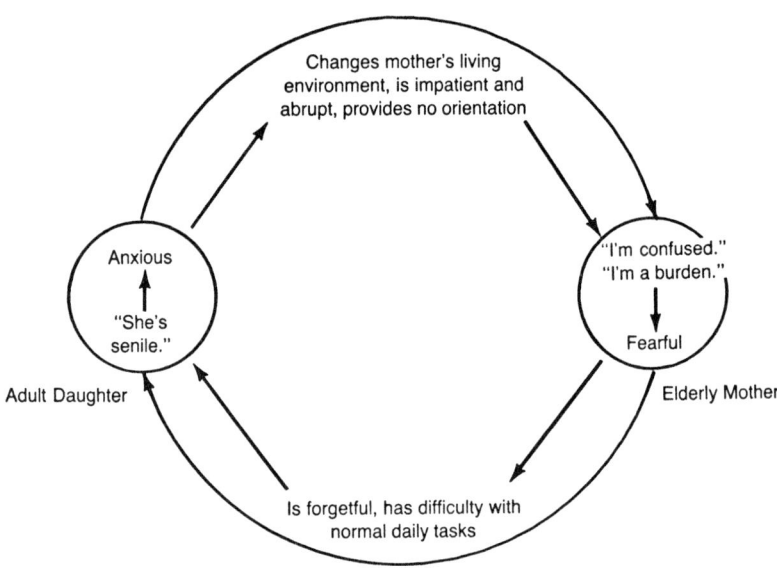

from sitting." The cycle continues as the son becomes increasingly aware of the complaints, attributing them to his father's old age (Figure 6–3).

The way in which the attempted solution to a problem perpetuates the problem instead of solving it is striking. Diagramming the vicious cycles of family interaction that affect and are affected by the problems of aging assists the professional in identifying new connections to "old" problems. An awareness of the cybernetic effect allows the therapist to see how "small but strategic changes, whose effects will be reinforced by interaction within the system, can interrupt the vicious cycles" (Herr & Weakland, 1979, pp. 52–53).

Case Example

A family was self-referred to the Family Nursing Unit,* Faculty of Nursing, University of Calgary, because of the 72-year-old maternal

---

*We are grateful to Fabie Duhamel, R.N., M.N., University of Calgary, for her permission to document some of her work with this family.

Figure 6–3 Vicious Cycle: Hypochondriasis

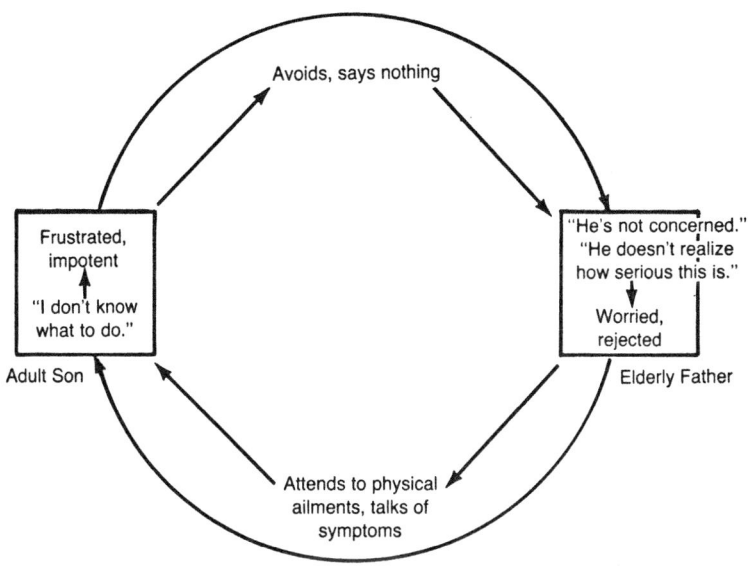

grandmother's "anxiety attacks" and refusal to get out of bed. At the time of referral, the household was composed of the mother, age 51, a part-time clerk in the husband's business; the father, age 50, self-employed; and the maternal grandmother (MGM), age 72. The couple had three daughters, aged 28, 24, and 20. The eldest two daughters were married, and the youngest daughter was attending college in another city. The maternal grandfather had died 4 years earlier of a coronary.

On the day of the first appointment, the mother called to cancel, stating that the MGM did not feel well enough to come to the Family Nursing Unit. It was decided to offer the family an appointment in their home and to use this important context change for the first interview as an opportunity to engage the MGM. To begin the engagement process, the therapist arranged the time for the home interview with the MGM. At the end of the first session in the home, the engagement of the family was evident by their agreement to have the second session at the Family Nursing Unit.

After a thorough family assessment by means of the Calgary family assessment model (Wright & Leahey, 1984), two problems were identified: (1) adjustment to a new living arrangement (whole family system problem) and (2) maladaptive interactional pattern between MGM and adult daughter (elderly parent-adult child system problem).

The MGM had relocated from another city to live with her eldest child and only daughter 2 months before the referral. This change in living arrangements was precipitated by the decision of the 46-year-old unmarried son (third child) to sell his mother's house. He felt that his mother was unable to continue living alone, since she had suffered a mild stroke. Though not involved in the decision to sell the house, the mother was asked to choose where she would like to live. She chose to live with her adult daughter, to whom she felt closest, even though this living arrangement constituted a move to another city.

The family assessment further revealed that the MGM presently felt rejected by both her sons and thought she was a burden to her adult daughter. She claimed, "I don't know where I belong or where to go." The adult daughter stated that she was willing for the MGM to live in her home as long as her mother behaved like a "healthy adult," which meant that the MGM be dressed, out of bed, and active each day. The son-in-law tended to be rather passive about the situation, which was hypothesized to be his way of avoiding triangulation between his wife and his mother-in-law.

Shortly after the MGM moved into her adult daughter's home, the daughter became frustrated with her mother's crying, complaining, and refusing to get out of bed. The daughter's reaction was to tell her elderly mother what to do in a rather bossy and demanding manner. The more demanding the adult daughter became, the more rejected and anxious the MGM became. Consequently, the MGM withdrew to her bed, crying and complaining. This, in turn, increased the adult daughter's frustration, thus continuing the vicious cycle. It is important to note that the onus of blame is *neither* with the elderly parent *nor* with the adult daughter; the problem is a relationship problem (Figure 6–4).

Recognizing the interrelationship of the two identified problems, the therapist hypothesized that the contributions of the MGM and those of her adult daughter to their interactional vicious cycle were attempts to control the other's behavior. Thus, the goal of the primary intervention was to break the maladaptive pattern and give *both* parties an opportunity to be in control. First, the therapist normalized the new joint living arrangement by noting that they were undergoing a major adjustment in living together as *adults*. The therapist stated that she was impressed with the caring and their desire to help one another.

The therapist prescribed an odd day/even day ritual (Selvini Palazzoli, Boscolo, Cecchin, & Prata, 1978) to enhance their caring and to interrupt the problematic cycle. The adult daughter was instructed to care for her mother (e.g., bring meals to her room) on the odd days of the week. On these days, the mother was to do as she pleased (e.g., stay in bed all

Figure 6–4 Vicious Cycle: Anxiety Attacks/Refusal to Get Out of Bed

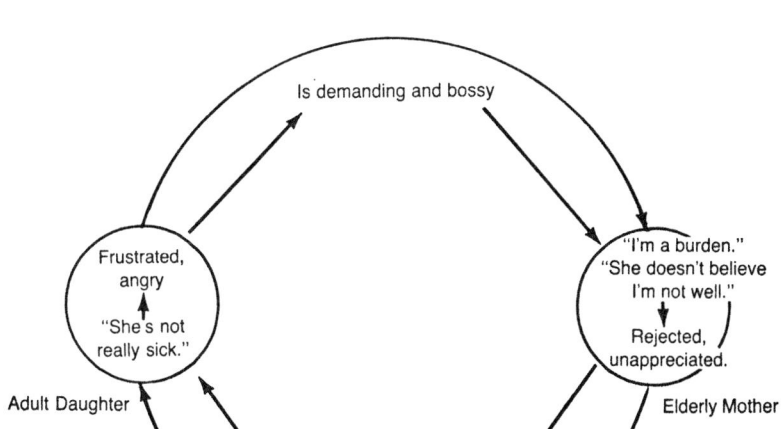

day). On the even days of the week, the MGM was to care for her daughter (e.g., help daughter make meals). On Sundays, they were to behave spontaneously. The intervention was well accepted, and the family members expressed relief and satisfaction both verbally and analogically.

By giving each member of the dyad permission to be in control of the caring expressed on alternate days, the intervention ritual interrupted the vicious cycle that had perpetuated the initial problems. The behavior of both parties and their perceptions of each other improved. The instruction for the adult daughter to bring meals to her mother interrupted her (the adult daughter's) bossy, demanding behavior, while the MGM's efforts to assist her daughter with meals required her (the MGM) to get out of bed. The caring behavior of each was positively perceived by the other. The MGM felt accepted and less anxious about where she belonged, and her bouts of crying were dramatically reduced. The adult daughter enjoyed having the assistance of her mother, which made it easier for her to reciprocate the expression of caring. Thus, an intergenerational virtuous cycle of caring was established (Figure 6–5).

86   FAMILIES WITH HANDICAPPED MEMBERS

Figure 6–5 Virtuous Cycle: Caring

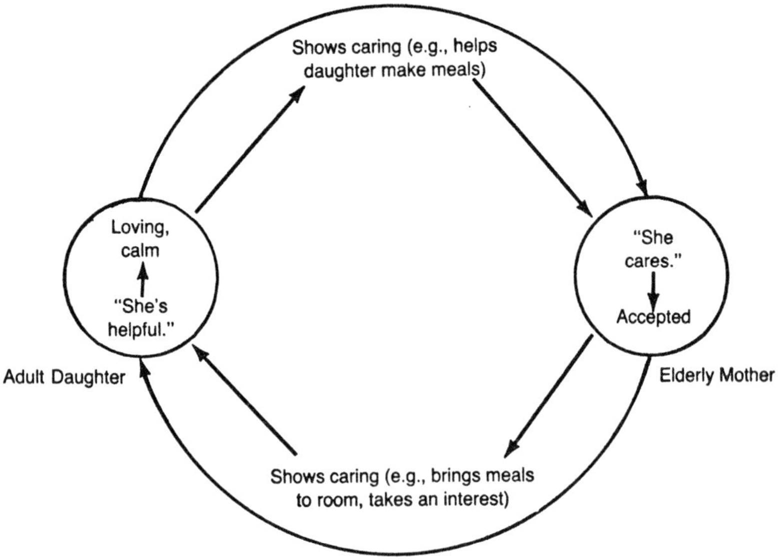

```
                    Shows caring (e.g., helps
                    daughter make meals)

      Loving,                                "She
       calm                                 cares."
        ↑                                      ↓
      "She's                                Accepted
      helpful."
   Adult Daughter                          Elderly Mother

                    Shows caring (e.g., brings meals
                    to room, takes an interest)
```

Since aging does not occur in a vacuum, it is most beneficial to consider the context within which an elderly person's concerns are arising. Failure to do so impedes a therapist's efforts to alleviate the handicapping symptoms. An interactional view of aging will help prevent the treatment of choice for an octogenarian from becoming "Take two tricyclic antidepressants and call the nursing home in the morning."

REFERENCES

Brody, E.M., & Kleban, M.H. (1983). Day-to-day mental and physical health symptoms of older people: A report on health logs. *The Gerontologist, 23*(1), 75–85.

Comfort, A. (1976). *A good age*. New York: Simon & Schuster.

Herr, J., & Weakland, J. (1979). *Counseling elders and their families*. New York: Springer.

Hirschfield, I.S., & Dennis, H. (1979). Perspectives. In P.K. Ragan (Ed.), *Aging parents*. Los Angeles: The Ethel Percy Andrus Gerontology Center, University of Southern California Press.

Kaplan, B.H. (1979). An overview of interventions to meet the needs of aging parents and their families. In P.K. Ragan (Ed.), *Aging parents*. Los Angeles: Ethel Percy Andrus Gerontology Center, University of Southern California Press.

Kramer, C.J., & Kramer, J.R. (1976). *Basic principles of long-term patient care*. Springfield, IL: Charles C Thomas.

Lieberman, G.L. Children of the elderly as natural helpers: Some demographic variables. (1978). In J.C. Glidewell & M.A. Lieberman, *American Journal of Community Psychology* [Special Issue], 6(5), 489–498.

Robinson, B., & Thurnher, M. (1979). Taking care of aged parents: A family cycle transition. *The Gerontologist*, 19, 586–593.

Selvini Palazzoli, M., Boscolo, L., Cecchin, G., & Prata, G. (1978). A ritualized prescription in family therapy: Odd days and even days. *Journal of Marriage and Family Counseling*, 4(3), 3–9.

Silverstone, B., & Hyman, H.K. (1976). *You and your aging parent*. New York: Pantheon Books.

Simos, B.G. (1973). Adult children and their aging parents. *Social Work*, 18, 78–85.

Tomm, K. (1980). Towards a cybernetic-systems approach to family therapy. In D.S. Freeman (Ed.), *Perspectives on family therapy*. Vancouver, BC: Butterworths.

Wright, L.M., & Leahey, M. (1984). *Nurses and families: A guide to family assessment and intervention*. Philadelphia: F.A. Davis.

Zarit, S.H., Reever, K.E., & Bach-Peterson, J. (1980). Relatives of the impaired elderly: Correlates of feelings of burden. *The Gerontologist*, 20, 649–655.

7. Frames and Reframing

Steve de Shazer
Eve Lipchik

A MAN COMPLAINED TO PICASSO THAT HIS PORTRAIT OF GERTRUDE Stein did not look like her. According to Foss (1971),

> Picasso is said to have replied: "Never mind, it will." Once we have come to accept Picasso's way of seeing, have come to accept his rules of personality projection onto canvas (that linear sketches, for example, could be used to refer to things like subjects of portraits that were formerly represented by curved lines: Cubism), we too will in part see Miss Stein as Picasso drew her; interpret her, if you like, accordingly. We see the world accordingly as our existing conventions (categories, projection rules) enable us to see it. Believing is seeing (p. 235).

Frames (ways of seeing) and the labels attached to the frames dictate (to a greater or lesser extent) what we *can* see: our point of view determines (to some extent) what happens next. Conceptually this seems clear not only in art and in science but also in everyday life: frames and their labels affect paradigm induced expectations and enable us to articulate and measure the world. Any concrete "fact" can have several different labels implying different frames (Watzlawick, Weakland, and Fisch, 1974): a glass can be labeled as "half full" (generally seen as implying an optimistic way of seeing things) or the same glass can be labeled as "half empty" (a pessimistic view).

FRAMES AND REFRAMING

The strength of labels was clearly articulated by a client who began to describe her problem with these words: "I'm letting my handicap cripple me." A victim of polio at a young age, she wore leg braces and used a crutch to aid her walking, and she believed she had adjusted to her handicap (since she knew nothing else). However, she was repulsed by the type of men who were attracted to her and thought that her handicap prevented her from ever having a chance for a relationship with a man she would find attractive. At the start of therapy she described herself as being depressed about her handicap for the first time in her life. In looking at herself the way she thought others saw her, she compared herself to other good-looking women her age and, at this point, found herself lacking. So, she started to make efforts to hide her handicap by placing the crutch out of sight, whenever possible.

The major focus of intervention in this case was the client's crutch and her efforts to hide it (de Shazer, 1979). Once she started to use canes that were unusual in design, color or shape *and* once she started to display these openly, she projected an unusual amount of strength. This made an impression on people which resulted in their treating her differently. Subsequently, she was also able to attract the kind of man she desired. As she put it during the last session, "I am no longer letting my handicap cripple me."

Her self-induced label of "cripple" helped to determine her approach to people and situations just as the new label, or frame, of "strength" helped to promote a new and different approach. Since the new frame elicited and promoted more rewarding responses she was able to maintain it.

This example points out the "looking glass" or interactional nature of frames and their labels. The client saw other people seeing her as crippled, adopted the label, and started to behave as if crippled. The more she behaved as crippled (for instance, placing her crutch out of sight as much as possible), the more people would see her as crippled, and the vicious cycle continued to maintain itself. When she started to exhibit stronger behavior (for instance, keeping her cane in open view), others saw her as strong, and she started to see them see her as strong, and the virtuous cycle began to maintain itself. Importantly, the change in labels can "start" anywhere in the system, so to speak. If others had started to see her as strong before she had seen herself in such a way, then they might have initiated the "strong frame" for her. Of course, in therapy, initiating the new frame was the task of the therapist, and there is a need for the therapist to be reasonably sure that the new frame will be reinforced by others.

CASE EXAMPLE

The therapy described in the following case was done at the Brief Family Therapy Center where a team approach is part of the standard operation. One member of the team is in the room with the clients while one or more are behind the mirror. After about 30 to 40 minutes of a session, the conductor of the session joins the rest of the team for a consulting break during which the major intervention message is designed. The therapist then returns to the room to deliver the message.

The following case is an application of an interactional understanding of frames and their associated labels and, therefore, an interactional view of the process of changing frames and labels based, at least in part, on a generalization of the process described in the above case. In this example, the frame had a life-threatening effect, and only the competent assessment of the referring social worker at the nursing home prevented a possible untimely death.

Mr. B was a 72-year-old white male who had been residing in a nursing home for the past six years. His permanent placement there occurred a year or so after he had suffered a stroke. At that time bladder problems and a broken hip made it impossible for his wife to care for him any longer in the home. Although the nursing home staff felt that his adjustment to the home had not been as good as it could be, in terms of his acceptance of his disability and some family tension, the patient's physical condition had been satisfactory and stable.

Two months prior to the initial appointment for family therapy, Mr. B had had an unexplained fall which left him very frightened and with some continuing pain. While the doctors at first considered the possibility that the fall had been caused by another mild stroke, or that Mr. B had had a temporary black-out for a variety of reasons, they later concluded that there was no physiological reason for his not having recovered the level of his previous functioning. His condition became increasingly worse: He lost 21 pounds by refusing to eat solid foods; he refused to get out of bed and to have any physical therapy; he lost interest in former activities (such as watching ball games); he became irritable and rejecting of the nursing home staff and, in particular, demanded the constant presence of his wife.

Prior to this, Mrs. B, who still worked full-time, would visit her husband in the evenings and on weekends, on a regular basis, except when she was too tired or had other plans. On those occasions, he had been accepting of this as long as he had been told in advance.

Since the unexplained fall, Mr. B demanded Mrs. B's daily presence and refused to let the staff do anything for him, waiting instead for the evening when he insisted Mrs. B do it all. At first Mrs. B complied, thinking that her compliance would speed her husband's recovery, but he seemed to get progressively worse and the more she tried to please him the more demanding and irritable he became. At this point she felt totally controlled not only by him, but also by the nursing home staff. If she did not visit daily and do all the things he demanded, he was not only angry with her but made trouble for the staff. The staff, in turn, complained to her and made her feel guilty. Since she was about to retire and was afraid her husband would demand even her daytime hours, she agreed to some family counseling.

The arrangements that were made for the first session were that Mrs. B would come by herself and Mr. B would be brought by a special wheelchair van. Mr. B appeared to be extremely angry from the start of the session. He denied having been told the purpose of the meeting and when he was informed of its reason his reply was: "Are things that bad?" He rejected all attempts by the therapist (Eve Lipchik) to establish any rapport with him, and whenever he did not like what he heard, he removed his hearing aid and wheeled himself away from her and his wife. Furthermore, the therapist was prevented from taking a one-down position with respect to Mr. B's unwillingness to participate by Mrs. B's urgent insistence that her husband make use of the session to talk and listen and her anger at his refusal to do so.

(Behind the screen, it seemed clear that Mr. B was a tough old s.o.b. who was discouraged and angry about his helplessness *and* dependence. When this idea was phoned in, and relayed to him by the therapist, he became more animated than at any other point in the session. He denied being a tough s.o.b. any longer, removed the hearing aid and wheeled himself away. Mrs. B, however, agreed that she had seen him as being a tough old s.o.b. prior to the fall. At this point, the team (Steve de Shazer, Insoo Berg, and Marilyn Bonjean) speculated that although Mr. B made demands, the compliance made him angry and confirmed his fears of being terminally ill. Therefore, if people were to stop giving in to his demands, it might prove to him that he could do things for himself again and he might become less angry.

(The team decided to establish a separate working alliance with Mrs. B before having another session with the couple. We thought that more information about the old pattern(s) would be useful. The following message was delivered after the whole team met for a consulting break.)

Intervention Message

Jonathan, we are very impressed with how difficult it must be for you to have to put up with all this, and not be with Judith all the time, but despite all that, you show a lot of spirit. You still look like a man who knows what he wants and you haven't given up. You still have a lot of spirit.

We are also impressed that after 42 years of marriage you still care for your wife so much.

Judith, we are also struck with your efforts to make Jonathan happy and still have a life of your own. Most wives would not be nearly as caring and loyal as you are.

We think you are both in a difficult situation, and the fact that you, Judith, are trying the best you can for *both* of you—not only yourself—is very impressive. Many women would not be so unselfish.

We would like to see you each, separately, for at least one session.

Mrs. B's attitude had changed somewhat when she returned the following week. She appeared less helpless and spoke of becoming tougher, even though "that was not her nature." She described Mr. B as having been a very proud, independent man who never asked for anything and who always tried to help others. Their relationship had been a good one of give and take. She illustrated this by relating how her husband had assumed some household duties when she went to work after the children got older, and how, when he did not like the way she cooked his eggs, or made his sandwiches for lunch, he simply took over making them the way he liked. This type of issue had never caused any hard feelings between them.

His illness and confinement to the nursing home had been a difficult adjustment for both of them, but she thought things had been tolerable until Mr. B's recent fall. She feared his changed behavior and steady decline were either a sign that the doctors were missing something and he was sicker than they thought, or that he had given up. She described dreading her visits with him not only because he was so demanding, but because the staff was so irritated with her for not making him behave better.

(During the consulting break, we decided to continue to work with Mrs. B alone for a while since she was already showing signs of changing.)

Intervention Message

We are impressed with what a good person you are—trying to help not only your sick husband but also the nursing home staff. We are also struck with how sensitive you are to other people's feelings. It seems that you don't want anyone else to hurt as much as you do, and will go to no end to try to make things better for them, even if it hurts you more.

From what you tell us, we can see that your husband was always a very independent man who took pride in being needed and helping his family. It must be hard for him to feel more and more reliant on others. On the other hand, it occurred to us that the more you try to help him by doing what he asks of you, the more dependent and helpless he must feel—and the less like his old self he can be—and the more irritable and hopeless he may get.

We have an idea that before he can give you more freedom, he will have to feel better about himself, and become more independent. In order to help him do that, you may have to sacrifice some of your usual helpful ways to make him feel needed by you, in some way, when you are with him. Your husband needs a challenge, like proving he can still do something for *you*, and therefore needs to see you as needing help in some way. You may even have to *pretend* to act sick or helpless or dependent to get him to help you. We know that this may be very hard for you and that you may not be able to do it at all, but we'd like you to go home and think about it.

One week later, Mrs. B reported that her husband had had a very good week. For the first time in months he was hungry and was eating solid food again. He had also agreed to go back to physical therapy and was working hard to regain his mobility. She did not really know how to account for these changes. However, she did describe a change in her attitude. His behavior during the first session made her decide that if the two of them were not going to be able to get help from therapy because of his behavior, she was just going to have to get tougher and live her own life even if it upsets him and the staff. She had told her husband that since he would not cooperate in therapy, she was going to go alone and get help for herself.

She also reported that she had stopped giving in to him so much this week. When he did not want to sit in the dining room with her while she had some coffee, she told him to go back to his room alone, and she would see him later. He did. She had decided that it was time to stop treating him like he was hopelessly ill and to stand up to him again, *which was her old pattern*. Her husband seemed a little surprised at her behavior this week, but was not complaining too much about it.

Intervention Message

We are glad things are better and that your husband is eating again, and more his old self, and that you have decided to, Judith, think about yourself more regardless of what Jonathan and the staff say to you.

It is quite understandable that when he got ill two months ago it was a shock, and you were afraid that he was dying, or would become totally helpless. Naturally, you responded by showing concern, by coming to see him more, and by giving in to all his demands to make him feel more comfortable and happy. We have a sense that he, too, feared the same things and that the more attention you gave him, the more his fears were confirmed.

Now, your decision to get counseling for yourself so you can lead your own life again, and to no longer give in to his every demand, is proving to him you see him as his old self, and no longer hopelessly ill. Continue proving to Jonathan you need to take care of yourself and that you feel that he is recovering.

Mrs. B came back two weeks later reporting that her husband was back to normal and doing very well. He was hungry all the time, had been gaining weight, and was ambulatory again. She did not visit daily and he did not complain about it. She had made plans to go on a weekend trip when her granddaughter graduated, and to spend a week at a lake in the summer. Her husband had gotten his sense of humor back and was enjoying his old activities. She spoke about her husband always having had both an "inferiority complex" and a sense of being very powerful. She illustrated this by relating how, whenever his favorite team lost, he would say: "I'm the jinx. They lost because I was listening." This made her think that he must also feel responsible for *her bad moods*, so when she does what is best for her and she is happier, it makes him feel better about himself. Even when pushed, she insisted that if her husband should get demanding again, she would continue to take time for herself and lead her own life for his sake, too. She now felt giving in to him only makes things worse.

(Since things were going so well, the team decided to terminate at this point.)

Intervention Message

Glad things are going so well. Sounds like Jonathan can really take care of himself again and is taking charge of his own recovery. We are pleased you are taking better care of yourself too, and not feeling so guilty about it. We agree with you that Jonathan seems to get a really good feeling about himself when he sees you are more your old self. It is probably the familiar feeling of being useful to you, of doing his part to help you feel good.

Occasionally, he may go through that little song and dance again about being a burden, but we feel that this is only his way of making sure you still care, and that you need him, too.

We're thinking that the best way for you to deal with Jonathan under all circumstances, even if he should get difficult or even sick again, is to treat him as much as possible like you did before he ever got sick.

The nursing home staff reports excellent physical recovery and that Mr. B's emotional adjustment is as good or better than before the fall.

DISCUSSION

Before the fall, Mr. B acted like, and was treated like, a proud, independent man who never asked for anything and tried to help others. This frame was shared by Mr. and Mrs. B and (within the limits of the situation) the staff of the nursing home.

After the fall, Mrs. B and the staff labeled their giving in to Mr. B's demands as "helpful," which implied they were operating within a frame describing Mr. B as "helpless," no longer strong, and no longer independent. The more they tried to be helpful, the more Mr. B labeled himself as "helpless," since this confirmed his frame which was built on his fears and his temporarily weakened physical condition. He came to believe he was helpless, and so stopped eating and confined himself to his bed to die. The less he ate and the less he moved, the weaker he got; and the more "helpful" people got, the more his worse fears were confirmed.

Thus the two labels, helpless and helpful, can be seen to interact to the detriment of all. The behaviors falling under each label tend to confirm the other label and a mutually escalating pattern develops.

Beginning in the first session, the therapy team aimed at changing these two labels. In spite of Mr. B's denials, when he was angry he could take action, like removing his hearing aid and wheeling himself around—much as he did before. His demonstration of this independence and the fact that there were no physical reasons for his increased helplessness, gave the team the clues for the development of an effective series of interventions.

CONCLUSION

The looking-glass nature of frames and their related labels suggested by the two problems and the therapeutic solutions, offers some idea about their power to determine what happens next and what is seen to happen. Furthermore, labels have an interactive relationship, as the second case illustrates. Recursively, the more "helpful" people became, the more "helpless" the patient became and this led to even more "helpful" behavior, etc. Handicaps can cripple, but they can also show strength, and the difference is far from trivial. In both cases, therapy provided a different type of mirror which helped people to *see* the situations differently and, thus, behave differently. The therapeutic shift, or reframing, from "cripple" to "strong," promoted a different enough difference in the clients' everyday interactions with others.

Even though two (or more) labels can be applied to the same situation, all labels are not equal. Some labels (and the frames that are implied) promote detrimental behavior while others promote beneficial behavior. Because labels are generalizations they distort situations by simplification. Consequently, part of the therapeutic task is to provide a mirror-image of the label, a different label which distorts in a more beneficial or nonproblematic direction for the purpose of promoting more useful behavior.

REFERENCES

de Shazer, S. (1979). On transforming symptoms: An approach to an Erickson procedure. *AJCH*, *22*(1), 17–28.

Foss, L. (1971). Art as cognitive: Beyond scientific realism. *Philosophy of Science*, *38*, 234–250.

Watzlawick, P., Weakland, J., & Fisch, R. (1974). *Change*. New York: Norton.

8. Mobilization: A Natural Resource of the Family

Sam Scott

According to Webster's *Seventh New Collegiate Dictionary*, the military definition of the term *mobilize* is to assemble and make ready for use as resources. All families have resources that can be either mobilized or immobilized by a traumatic event. The family that learns one of its members is disabled mobilizes not only around the disability per se, but also along several other fronts. Family members mobilize to defend what they consider to be a vulnerable spot in the family. They mobilize to initiate actions that will organize the family into a unit. The family mobilizes to ask questions and gather information from the doctors and hospitals, family members, and friends. This is a normal process.

THERAPIST'S ROLE

To discover what resources are available, the therapist must hear and accept the family's own way of coping at the beginning of treatment. The therapist's use of the family's own vocabulary and acceptance of the family's self-image cement the bond of trust between the family and the therapist. Professionals at times try to mobilize a family based on their own assumptions of appropriate mobilization strategies. In so doing, they often neglect the family's existing mobilization tools. Naturally, not all means of mobilizing are adaptive and productive, but there are inevitably some positive means that the family employs and the therapist can use.

The therapist who is listening and responding must focus on the information given by family members. In other words, the therapist must focus on the concrete problem as it is presented by the family and, at the same time, deal with the issues that surround that problem. It is important to determine how the family uses its resources and how family members deal with the problems around the disability. Family members will tell the therapist very clearly how they perceive the problem, what it is, and what should be done about it. The therapist should make use of the way the family is dealing with the problem, since it is a way that makes sense to them.

The therapist must be sensitive to the family's emotional history. During pregnancy, parents look forward to the birth of a normal child. This frame of reference is a natural one. With the birth of a child, parents look forward to all the rewards that accompany such an event, e.g., regular visits from friends and relatives, gifts to celebrate the birth, and compliments on their child. They begin to discuss schools and education, and to look around the neighborhood to see if there will be other children the same age as their child. The dream is shattered by the birth of a handicapped child. Even if the handicap was suspected in advance, a psychological disruption has taken place in the family. In place of happy expectations are disillusionment, fear, and isolation. Each family member must confront the diagnosis. The therapist who is truly listening will feel the shock waves that emanate from a family that has been so traumatized. Each family member, indeed the whole family, should believe that someone understands their plight. The therapist may have to deal with rage, anger, depression, or guilt as the parents realize that they have a handicapped child.

How long does it take to work on rage, anger, depression, or guilt? What can or should be done? One answer is to work on the problems the family presents and, if these feelings arise, deal with them. A great deal of energy goes into rage, anger, depression, and guilt. The therapist can make this energy positive by using it to help mobilize the family in a productive way. It is important to remember that the family with a problem has already mobilized positive elements by seeking therapy.

FAMILY #1

The following is a history and transcript of an interview with a family whose members considered themselves a normal family with a handicapped child. It is an interview, not a therapeutic session. Professionals viewed the family as one that coped well with the trauma it faced.

Language

Since the language in the transcripts could be interpreted in a variety of ways, the author has delineated for discussion those parts of language that are read by the author as being positive. This will allow the reader to have a greater understanding of the language of mobilization as the author defines it. It will also illustrate the use of listening and responding in a specific way to the language the family presents.

Here is a note on language the author views as negative. When one considers the following elements of a mobilization response—overprotectiveness, guilt, denial, and the like—whoever is being talked about is placed in the position of needing help and the response is assumed to be negative. Sometimes these so called negative responses are adaptive at the time. It's when they subsequently prevent positive movement by the family that they become maladaptive. As therapists know, there is a vast difference between one who expresses a need for help and one who is told he needs help. It is unfortunate that the term "overprotective" is utilized when parents of the disabled are seen. In fact, parents should be told, "you've pulled your resources together and you've mobilized the best way you could and it's not working for you." In therapy, what should be taking place is "What can therapists do to remobilize families in a direction that does work for them?"

Unfortunately, therapists look at the problems presented and compound them with the disability label and then add the label of guilt and overprotectiveness. Families are then required to deal with their anger and nonacceptance.

Therapists should focus on the concrete problem as it is presented by the family and at the same time deal with the issues that surround that problem.

Family History

At the time of the interview, the mother and father had been married about 7 years. They had a 6-year-old daughter who was not handicapped, but their 3-year-old son had several congenital defects, including a cleft lip and palate, a heart problem, and a respiratory problem. In addition, he had seizures and a chemical imbalance. At the time of the interview, he had been admitted to the hospital 12 times. There were hospital admissions for plastic surgery to repair the lip and palate, for bronchitis, and for respiratory distress. He had also been admitted for several myringotomies. At the time of the interview, he also had acute intestinal problems. The physicians at first believed that the delay in the boy's development was due to the long and repetitious stays in the hospital, but 3 months before this interview, they told the parents that the boy was retarded.

Interview Transcript

Interviewer: And you all were recommended as one who coped well. Let's . . . you're Edward, and it's Ellen, is it? Ellen, let's start with that, let's start with the present. What are some of the problems that you see with the situation and you give us the diagnosis as you understand it. Start from that.

Mother: I guess the biggest problem is coping with the whole idea that he is retarded. We were given the diagnosis that he was laterally retarded. Our feeling is that we are not taking all of what we've heard at face value. We feel the children are very hard to judge to begin with and, although we know we have the problem, we are, we're

going to do our damndest to prove them wrong. So we are adjusting, and we've adjusted to the problem that he does not present a problem.
Interviewer: What are the greatest difficulties that you see right now?
Mother: Right now, just accepting it.
Interviewer: How does one do that?
Mother: I don't know if anyone ever accepts it completely.

It would be easy to demonstrate that the preceding transcript is filled with nonacceptance and an inability to adjust. Because the family has adjudged itself normal, however, the conversation can be perceived in a different way. The statement that the "biggest problem is coping and the whole idea that he's retarded" could distance the mother from her child's retardation. Although the statement could be considered denial, the "idea" represents a more accurate statement of the mother's feelings about labeling.

There are several different kinds of denial. For example, denial can be productive or malproductive. The conviction with which the mother says "our damndest to prove them wrong" following the common sense statement that "children are very hard to judge" is very positive in that it allows the parent to look forward to a future time. The mother is saying, "You, the professional, are not sure, so I'm not buying." Naturally, there must be a time frame associated with this comment. Such a comment is appropriate after early contacts with diagnosing professionals, but they can be nonproductive or malproductive later. The goal is to direct the parents' energy into an activity that helps them work with the child to help him reach his fullest potential. From this point of view, the preceding transcript quote had the quality of "Damn the torpedoes"—a real case for mobilization.

The phrase "given the diagnosis" could be interpreted as the mother's denial, but it is also a statement of the physician's belief, not her own. "We've heard at face value" could be interpreted to mean that the parents are ready for physician/hospital shopping; it could also be looked at as a wait-and-see position. The statement "we know we have a problem" indicates that the parents are in touch with the reality of the situation, but are resisting the label. Saying "to prove them wrong" could be interpreted as a rejection of the physicians, the label, or the implications of the label (e.g., limitations on development, capacity for speech). If the last interpretation is more to the point, it might mean that extra effort could realistically bring about better results than the physicians predict. This level of denial is usually the cornerstone of a productive approach to the difficulty.

The father was asked about a grieving process—loss of the normal child. He was asked how he responded when he was informed of the boy's congenital defects.

> Father: When he was first born. My own feelings, I felt like I really got kicked in the face. Why did that happen to me? But there's no answer to that. I felt this enormous initial sense of shock, and then I just kinda', I felt like I was down on the ground and I said to myself, "Well, being down on the ground is not going to help matters at all, let alone my son. I'm going to pick myself up, and I'm going to just do whatever I can for myself, for Ellen. You know being weak is not going to help in a situation like that. I know I just have to be strong and kinda' pull my life together."

One way of interpreting this section of the transcript is to say that the father is asserting that the problem is something he can personally control and is refusing to admit helplessness. On the other hand, he could be talking about how he will cope with the problem, rising above the "fight or flight" response. In this situation, there is nothing to fight and nothing from which to take flight. In addition, the father responded naturally. "I felt like I really got kicked in the face."

The mother was also asked about the grieving process.

> Mother: I went through a really bad time when he was first born. I even had trouble getting out of bed for a few weeks. It was just a total shock; I just couldn't handle any of it until we were allowed to see him. He was about a month old. And for some reason he was my baby that was [unintelligible] of it. Then I just starting coming around and then when we found out he was retarded.... There are times when I look at, I never try to compare him to somebody else his age. There are times now, of course, when I see a little boy his age, and I get very upset.
>
> Father: That bothers me too.
>
> Mother: We have good days and bad days. I know this, some days I'm really bad, and I know that it's OK 'cause tomorrow or the next day I'll feel better. There are days when I'm fine. There are days when I'm great.

Interviewer: Do both of you take that attitude that the depression that you might feel will go away?
Father: Oh yeah, absolutely.

The exchange "when I see a little boy his age, and I get very upset." "That bothers me, too." could be interpreted to indicate unresolved envy, but it could mean that the parents are facing reality with less and less difficulty.

Since family history is important, it is natural to discuss the reactions of the grandparents to the birth of a disabled child. The couple was asked about the responses of other family members.

Father: Extremely supportive.
Interviewer: How, what happened?
Father: They just let us know that they understood and they'll support us.
Mother: Do you mean what they said when we told them?
Interviewer: If you can think of anything, sure, when you told them.
Mother: My mother said, "Well, I'm glad we finally know so that we can get him into a school and get him the help that he needs." And my mother-in-law said nothing. Not too much, she . . .
Father: I think she was maybe a little shocked, and perhaps she didn't want to say the wrong thing, so she really didn't say a whole lot. My mother's the kind of person that nothing really bothers her . . .
Mother: Yeah, she looked at our son and said, "Look at him, he looks so bright, look what he's doing, isn't that fabulous. Oh, he's so cute, he's so smart, he's so great."

The comment "Well, I'm glad we finally know so that we can get him . . . the help that he needs." is a thoughtful and articulated statement of support that admits there is a problem. In interpreting "Oh, he's so cute, he's so smart, he's so great." as a statement of denial, it should be noted that the mother remembered the statement and clearly understood that her mother-in-law was denying in a nonproductive way.

As is the case with many families that have a disabled member, it is difficult to attend to individual and couple needs. In many instances, attending to those needs seems next to impossible. It is crucial to determine if the denial is dysfunctional and if the family is in pain over it.

Interviewer: When you all go out, who takes care of the kids?
Father: Well, I'll let Ellen tell . . .
Mother: You mean when Eddie and I go out? We have a sitter, a program sitter.
Father: She's like a member of the family.
Interviewer: Is she an older person?
Mother: No, she's a girl; she's a teen-ager.
Interviewer: And she's able to handle your son?
Mother: . . . I spent 2 or 3 weeks at home training her on how to take care of our son, and then she took care of him. . . . We don't just call anybody; we have somebody specific. And then, of course, my mother or his parents will sit if we need them.

The remarks about "training her to take care of our son" and "We have somebody specific." are clear, concrete evidence that they acknowledge their son's problems. The parents take a responsible attitude toward their son's problems, while protecting the needs of the couple. This family has worked out a system that utilizes the extended family and carefully selected and trained sitters. This is mobilization.

FAMILY #2

The following family has mobilized in a way that has not been successful.

The family consisted of the mother and father, Michael, a 21-year-old sister, and a 19-year-old brother. Both siblings were attending college and were ostensibly out of the home. At the time the family was seen, Michael, the identified patient, was 24 years old. The parents believed that they had been unsuccessful in their dealings with psychiatrists, social workers, and psychologists over the last 22 years. Throughout the life of this young man, the people in social services had been telling the parents that it was their responsibility to separate from their son, that it was their responsibility to become less involved. The immediate problem was acting out behavior, e.g., hitting mother, and behavior problems at the workshop.

The young man was very dependent on his parents, who washed him, cut up his food, and demanded little of him in the way of chores. He had been born with hydrocephalus, which was alleviated by a shunt. The parents were told he would be retarded. Although he had an IQ of 90, he was in the lowest section of a sheltered workshop for the retarded. Until recently, his mother had bathed him and seen to his toilet needs. He had not poured a glass of milk until recently. He was not allowed to walk outside the house unsupervised; he was not allowed to go to work by himself.

The family came to the clinic nine times over a period of a year and a half. The issues worked on were very concrete, and the family was expected to practice. Therapy was intended to remobilize the family in a direction that was more beneficial. Although there were obvious marital conflicts (the couple had been married for 35 years), the goal with the parents was to resolve parental issues.

The following is a transcript of the first therapy session with this family.

> Therapist: I know about some of the problems, but suppose you tell me what the problem stems from, and where it comes from and what goes on.
>
> Mother: I don't know exactly, but there are times when he comes home and he's very, very angry and he won't talk about it immediately, you know. Maybe he'll wait and some little something will happen around the house—an incidental little thing that doesn't mean anything—and suddenly he flares up because of something that happened last week.

It is easy to conclude from the preceding transcript that the mother is minimizing the importance of the incidents that have taken place. The son's behavior is presented as bizarre and unprovoked. The mother has removed herself from responsibility for them, since her presentation of the incidents implies that the son's behavior is totally undiscriminating. Another way of listening to the information presented by the mother is to accept and believe what she is saying from her perception. At the same time, the responding therapist takes therapeutic control by narrowing down the information offered.

> Therapist: What does the flare-up consist of?
> Mother: Oh, he actually swings . . .
> Therapist: You?
> Mother: At anybody near him.
> Therapist: You?
> Mother: Yeah, me—anybody, doesn't matter to him.
> Therapist: He hits you?
> Mother: Oh he has . . . of course, he misses many times, too.

Therapist: But he has hit you, huh?
Mother: Oh yeah . . .
Therapist: Before we get away from that, I'd like to stay with it just a moment because it's disturbing obviously.
Mother: Yes, it is.
Therapist: When he hits you, on the occasions that he has hit you, what have you done?
Mother: I hit him back . . . but he's not allowed to touch mother.
Therapist: How does that work when you hit him?
Mother: Well, he'll take his punishment, but he's glad he did it.

The narrowing down of the mother's information is effective for several reasons. It allows the mother to realize that someone is listening to her plight, because the questions are a response to her original statement. It shows that someone is willing to pursue the topic without making a judgment and without quickly asking her what part she played in the son's behavior. The therapist's repetition of what was being done to her surprised the mother and conveyed the idea that this was a significant event not to be tolerated. If the mother were asked to admit that she played a part, she could hardly trust the therapist.

The following is the father's answer when the therapist asked him what he saw as being the problem.

Father: To relate to the tension that he might be coming home with, where it's been with him so long, that we can realize it when it happens, then it could be an offshoot of a remark, is relative to a remark said in his place of work in this respect: "Well, that's just what so and so did" (and he names the person), and I say, "Well why do you think he did it?" "He gave no reason for doing it." I say, "Well, when was it done? (Answer: "When the supervisor was not there.") So I says, "Well, when the supervisor came, what happened?" (Answer: "Everybody was at attention. Everyone was quiet.") And I said, "Well, what happened to you?" (Answer: "Then I was angry.") So he would flip a chair at the person. He does not have the presence of mind, I feel, to control it. He'll do it later, but it's more of a delaying action type of anger and frustration. Secondly, when they issue edicts, this is most pronounced, of taking things from the floor because a person might fall. This is, he takes to the

> highest degree, so much so he picks up paper and he has, he will not permit anyone to lure him away from this object that he takes, whether it be paper or anything from the floor, even if it's so much as a counselor beating him bodily and saying "Get to your place of work." He says, "Someone might trip, and I cannot take back an injury."
>
> Therapist: Do you see that as a problem?
> Father: That's a big problem, because, now he is going to the men's room and washing the floor because they might slip, and then people fall over him and they push him. This is the aggravation for me because they see him crouched in a position and the tendency is to push him over.

One way of looking at the father's description is that it is literal, obsessive, narrow, and without a sense of proportion. A therapist could deal with each of the elements and spend hours discussing the meanings. This man has lived with a difficult problem for many, many years. He and his family have gone from therapist to therapist. It took many years and many therapists to train the father to offer such obsessive detail to get to "they push him." In saying "They push him," the father is actually saying, "They push him, and it hurts me." In all of what the father said, the core of his feeling is his worry about his son. To create a sense of trust in the father, the therapist need only attend to the father's worry about his son. Once that concern is attended to, the parents of this young man have sufficient trust in the therapist to permit successful therapy.

The following is a transcript of a therapeutic intervention with the same family. The father needed to be in control of the son. The therapist made use of the compulsive and repetitive behavior of the father by directing him to deal with his son in a compulsive and repetitive way. For example, the son had a habit of turning off the TV during the evening news. The father was asked if that was acceptable to him. He answered, "No." The therapist pressed the father for a response. The father finally said he would dismiss the young man from the room.

> Father: If you go out of the room while I listen to the news.
> Son: No, because you'll just turn it on the next day, Monday morning.
> Father: (*confused*) I'll turn it on Monday morning, for what?

Therapist: Don't get carried away by the next conversation, John. You are dealing with the evening news right now, and that's it.
Father: Just the evening news.
Son: And I said no, because you might get carried away and do it Monday morning.
Father: Well, then you're going to stay out of the room.
Son: No! I'm going to turn it off and watch something else. I've done it before, and I'll do it again.
Father: Well, I'll force you to stay out of the room.
Son: I'm not going to be forced to watch it. I'll either turn it off and turn something else on and sit there and that's it. I'm not going to . . .
Father: No! I'll force you to stay out of the room.
Son: You're not going to force nothing. You just leave me alone and let the program alone. I'm not wearing out the set.
Father: Wearing out the set? That has nothing to do with it. I'll have to force you to stay out.

In the first session, family members were accepted as they were, with little or no direction. The preceding transcript, however, shows that directives in succeeding weeks became activity-oriented. Family members followed direction week after week. Just as repetition ennobled the parent's difficulties, the repetition of directives week after week created a tighter bond between the therapist and the family.

The family not only followed directives, but also modeled some of the therapist's behaviors, even using some of the therapist's words. It was no different from the therapist's use of the words the family used in the beginning session. Each member trusted the therapist to handle his or her vulnerability with understanding.

CONCLUSION

Each family has its own characteristics. There are different ways of listening and responding to the information presented by a family. In these cases, the listening provided the frame of reference for positive mobilization and allowed the therapist to respond with understanding. The listening and responding to the language of mobilization encouraged the family to endure the stress of change. It is important to be aware of the family's ability to mobilize, of the difficulties they have faced, and of their need to be considered a well family, a good family. Responding to the information with respect in the beginning session gives handsome rewards to the therapist in later sessions.

9. A Social Action Perspective: The Disabled and Their Families in Context

Laurie MacKinnon
Nancy Marlett

The meaning of the term *handicapped* has been seriously challenged by a growing number of disabled adults. They maintain that their difficulties reflect not their biological limitations, but the discrimination that prevents them from entering the mainstream of society. Like the civil rights activists of other minorities, physically disabled adults have created independent organizations to assert their rights of self-determination and access to social and employment opportunities (Bowe, 1978; Heumann, 1979; Hourihin, 1979).

These groups have made major headway in securing access to full participation in community life. Transportation for the disabled, access to buildings and public transportation, nondiscriminatory hiring contract clauses, and independent living support networks are but a few of the advances made. The emergent power of self-help crystallized in centers for independent living across North America. In these, disabled persons take responsibility for managing technical aides, home support, transportation, and congregate care, with professionals hired as consultants. The success of this movement has called into question societal and professional beliefs that the disabled are "unable" and attests to the value of focusing efforts outward toward social barriers rather than inward toward the specific problems of the disability.

This challenges current professional approaches, including family therapy, in which the distress of disabled persons and their families is considered inherent to the disability. Even when social factors are acknowledged, their implications for family therapy are generally ignored, and the therapist often retreats into the accepted practice of operating as if the problem required only some internal adjustment within the family. Inability of the family to adjust is then perceived to indicate deeper family dysfunction.

While it could be argued that family therapists do not intend to deal with social or political issues, the refusal to deal with the problem of disability as a social issue is, in itself, the taking of a political position. Furthermore, therapists who conceptualize the problem as inherent to either the disability or the family processes reinforce the family's perception of themselves as deviant, thereby encouraging the withdrawal, isolation, and helplessness of the family and the disabled person.

PARADIGMS OF SOCIAL PROBLEMS

The approach taken by the disability movement in externalizing and politicizing the causes of their difficulties falls within a social action paradigm that examines the differential distribution of society's resources, such as wealth, privilege, and political power. Social "problems" are, in fact, conflicts over the control of these resources and would not exist if the status quo were not to the economic and political advantage of certain groups within society (Rule, 1971). Change occurs primarily through the organization and political action of the minority group, not through the intervention of experts.

Current approaches to families with a disabled member do not fall within a social action paradigm, but rather emanate from a social pathology paradigm (Gliedman & Roth, 1980). Problems are defined as deviations from the accepted norms of behavior, and solutions are sought through objective assessment of the clinical, social policy, and research issues that concern the particular group requiring help. Such a paradigm, Gliedman and Roth (1980) stated, oversimplifies the problem of social change in the face of prejudice and social discrimination. The social pathology paradigm is perhaps most clearly reflected in the beliefs that professionals have evolved in the last three decades, many of which still prevail:

- Overprotection and idealization are used by parents to avoid the reality of the disability.
- Insistence on obtaining full information and services is "shopping around" for an alternate diagnosis in order to deny the reality of the handicap.
- Parental depression is the result of incomplete grief over the loss of the idealized child.
- Guilt, rage, and hostility are frequent dynamics in the family with a disabled member.
- Parents who cope successfully and remain optimistic are overcompensating to diminish their sense of guilt.
- Family dysfunction results from an inadequate emotional adjustment to bearing an "eternal child."

Similar notions can still be found in recent family therapy literature, and little or no attention is drawn to the social factors that maintain family difficulties (Bishop & Epstein, 1980; Ferrari, Mathews, & Barabas, 1983; Kaslow & Cooper, 1978; Leob, 1977; Shapiro & Harris, 1976; Turner, 1980; Woodard & Woodard, 1982).

Darling (1979) and others (Gliedman & Roth, 1980; Philp & Duckworth, 1982) challenge these beliefs, indicating that parents of normal children are actually more likely to idealize their child and to assess their child's abilities unrealistically. "Shopping around" occurs when professionals withhold information, give no support in the day-to-day realities, and offer a negative "victim blaming" view of the situation. While grief, guilt, rage, and hostility frequently emerge, they are not "natural" results of bearing a disabled child; the parents' reaction occurs in response to negative societal values and to the social barriers that will now exist for the family and the child. Approaches that strive only for psychological adjustment fail to acknowledge the ongoing social discrimination that makes true adjustment extremely difficult (Philp & Duckworth, 1982).

Within a social pathology paradigm, counseling is the solution prescribed for problems, since it is believed that people create their own difficulties (Darling, 1979). The attribution of responsibility to these families, often referred to as victim blaming, "only worsens their problems, and covertly legitimates the unnecessary suffering which many of the disabled and their families endure" (Philp & Duckworth, 1982, p. 106). Family therapy's basis in systems theory, because of its apparent neutrality and lack of content, covertly supports the fiction that families can be seen in isolation from social, economic, and political contexts (James & McIntyre, 1983). "To the extent that family therapists either deny or minimize the social content of family distress, and at the same time attribute to that family via their interventions, full responsibility for its 'dysfunction,' they participate in the reproduction of this fiction" (James & McIntyre, 1983, p. 124).

Clearly, any discussion of therapy with families that have a disabled member must include the current and historical relationship between these families and professionals. The "characteristics" attributed to the disabled and their families may be artifacts not only of the general social context, but also of the paradigm used by professionals in understanding the problem and interacting with the families. Of greater concern than the possibility that therapeutic interventions will be based on simple misperception is the possibility that these assumed characteristics will conflict between professionals and parents. When parents are defined as dysfunctional and thus in need of therapy because they do not cooperate with the plans of professionals, therapists may well be inadvertently involved in aspects of social control. To understand the circular nature of the therapist-family relationship, it is necessary to have a description of the events as perceived by the disabled and their families—the social action perspective.

THE CHANGING SOCIAL CLIMATE

The social context of families with a disabled member is complex. Furthermore, the social forces that affect a family with a disabled infant change markedly by the time the infant is an adult, and the family's style of coping formed during one era may be less effective in coping with the changed conditions of the next era. A sociohistorical perspective allows a therapist to view apparent dysfunction as the family's continuation of its response to the social forces operative when they first experienced the impact of the disability, even though those social forces have changed.

The disabled were first recognized as a unique group in the 1850s. Social attitudes at that time were remarkably similar to some current thinking in the rehabilitation field; the disabled were to be given the opportunity to develop to their full potential and to find a useful purpose within a controlled world (Kanner, 1964). This enlightened concern began to degenerate around 1870, however, and by 1890, the public attitude was one of pity and charity. A protective residential care model was developed, and increasing numbers of persons were permanently moved out of society to spare them the stresses of normal life (Kugel & Wolfensberger, 1976). Families were supported in their painful decision to place their child "away."

The science of eugenics later swept across America and Europe, alarming the public about the unchecked fertility of the "unfit" (Kanner, 1964). The mentally retarded began to be seen as a threat to society. Citizens pressed for the establishment of farm colonies because of the "great menace that the feeble minded are to the moral and social life of our communities, and to our public institutions, including the public schools" (Flanagan, 1970). The families of the mentally retarded were also ostracized and often broke contact with their retarded member in order to regain favor within the community. Inexpensive human warehouses were developed with little intent to promote growth and human dignity. The institutionalization approach was dominant from the 1920s into the 1980s and it is still a major service model today, despite the growing acceptance of normalization and deinstitutionalization (Marlett, 1978).

Families of the 1950s

In the 1950s, parents of retarded children began to rebel against forced institutionalization. Against the recommendations of professionals, some parents kept their children at home and fought to establish services in the community. Parents, particularly those of the 1950s and 1960s, described the responses of professionals as one of their greatest problems (Kratoville, 1975). They reported that information was deliberately withheld from them or delivered in an insensitive manner, that physicians often seemed unwilling to provide respectful care to the child, and that professionals seemed to blame them, particularly if they refused institutionalization (Darling, 1979). Therapists seemed oblivious to the parents' real concerns and undermined their confidence in raising their child (Kratoville, 1975).

In response to the unsupportive and hostile social climate, families formed rigid external boundaries, and parents joined with other parents of disabled children in developing a subculture that sought change through political action. Such collective action succeeded in improving the quality of community care for disabled children by establishing schools, workshops, group homes, and preschool programs.

The disabled children of the 1950s are now adults, and their families, although often weary from their earlier battles, are still blazing trails for better services. There are few opportunities for the disabled adult to live an independent, productive, and economically viable life. Where such opportunities do exist, parents often disagree with professionals over the young adult's future. Influenced by the disability movement, those currently in the field of rehabilitation propose that the disabled adult leave the family home to live "independently," i.e., in a setting controlled by an agent other than the family. Discussions between parents and professionals may be hindered by the parents' memory of earlier battles to keep their child at home. Their reluctance to have the disabled adult child leave the home is often the result of their unwillingness to relinquish ownership of the problem; the lesson of the previous era was that they could not trust outsiders. Professionals and parents may engage in extended debates over which of them has the responsibility, rather than allowing the disabled young adult to assume responsibility and working together to help the young person overcome obstacles to self-determination.

Not all families of the 1950s resist separation; some families are eager for the young person to assume more independence. The parents feel a sense of deep loss, however, when the separation occurs. They have foregone relationships within the community and sometimes with each other in order to cope with the pressures of raising their child. The disabled child not only has provided meaning and purpose to their lives, but also has often served as the basis for the parents' social contacts through relationships developed in the parents' movement. The "empty nest" is, therefore, experienced as a crisis until new networks are established. Within a social pathology paradigm, the family factors that impede separation may be conceptualized as overinvolvement of the mother, personality traits of the parents that inhibit the natural separation, or a marriage that is maintained by the disabled person's involvement. The fact that the family's rigid external boundary and the parents' "overinvolvement" were functional and necessary for the era in which the handicapped child was born is not always recognized.

Families of the 1960s

By the 1960s, parent-sponsored community services were being developed as an alternative to institutionalization. Parents began to rest easy, assuming that the services would continue. Although negative experiences with professionals were still commonplace, some parents, particularly those with physically disabled youngsters, were receiving more help from the medical community. However, the education system was still largely inadequate in preparing disabled children for an independent life style, and most parents believed that their child would never separate from the family.

The permanence of residence in the home is now being challenged, not only by professionals, but also by the disabled adolescents themselves, who now expect independence. The rebelliousness and disruption that ensue is often dramatically painful to the parents, who never anticipated such apparent "betrayal." Parents must also live with the unpredictability of their child's future. Where once, as they reached adulthood, mentally disabled persons moved from special schools to sheltered workshop settings, and physically disabled persons entered nursing homes; these alternatives are no longer predictable, however. Workshop settings have become overgrown and bureaucratized. Physically disabled persons object to the definition of physical disability as an illness and resist placement in nursing homes. Asserting that physical limitations should not abrogate a person's control over decisions that affect life events, disabled activists are pressing for services that will enable young people to establish themselves in the community, but such services are by no means secure or commonplace.

Families of the 1970s

In the 1970s, legislative mandates (e.g., P.L. 94-142) established the rights of disabled persons. Such legislation was enacted through the concerted efforts of parents, disabled persons, and a small emergent group of social action professionals (e.g., teachers, psychologists, social workers) who broke from established professional lines to advocate reform. The social climate was dramatically different from that of the 1950s, as professionals in social services began to accept responsibility for providing services to the disabled. As a result, the majority of families with disabled children born during the 1970s faced less severe deficits in services for their children and had less need to band together to fight the system. They formed fewer attachments to the subculture of the parents' organizations. Some parents' organizations report a "generation gap"; younger parents do not identify with the crusading stance taken by older parents and often withdraw from organizations.

Because of these differences, families of the 1970s face stresses not encountered by their predecessors. Families with a disabled member are still subject to stigma and discrimination. Without a subculture, they may feel more isolated, and the process of challenging social myths and arriving at a definition of themselves that is not victim blaming is inherently more difficult (Darling, 1979). Thus, the family is more vulnerable and may have greater difficulty in assuming a stance that challenges social norms.

With the disabled child's greater access to the mainstream, family members may more painfully experience stigma because the disabled member's presence in the community is more obvious. Siblings and the disabled child, for example, often attend the same school and must daily confront their differentness from other families. Integration is a circular process, influenced both by the degree of openness of the community to the family and child, and by the family's ability to reach out to their neighbors, educate them, and modify their usual response to pity, fear, and ostracism. Such an approach entails risk as the child moves into integrated settings. It also requires what families of the 1970s may lack—a solid alternate belief system and support network.

Families of the 1980s

Progress made prior to 1980 may now be jeopardized by a worldwide recession. "Reaganomics" in the United States and similar economic policies in Canada and other Western nations are severely eroding the social services and equal opportunities that the disabled and their families have struggled to obtain over the past 30 years. The Canadian province of British Columbia, for example, made headlines in 1983 by severely cutting support to disabled persons and simultaneously cutting back the Human Rights Commission.

Families with disabled children born in the late 1970s and 1980s are fighting a constant threat of cutbacks in medical treatments, technical aides, and in-home services. Only vigilant efforts by parents and social action professionals have prevented cutbacks in the funding of special education programs.

Older families may face another challenge as services that support disabled adults in the community are jeopardized. A government-imposed ceiling on rent subsidies in Alberta, for example, has forced some adults to return to a group home or institution because the rent on appropriately renovated apartments now exceeds the government's limits. Publicly supported transportation for disabled persons, the lifeline to participation in the community, is threatened whenever civic budgets are cut. Projects considered necessary to support recent gains have been postponed. The process of deinstitutionalization itself is at risk. In the long term, integration of the disabled into the community is less expensive; in the short term, however, costs are higher because of the need for specialized staff to assist in the relocation process. With the cutbacks, many institutions will be reduced to providing custodial care only and, therefore, will be unable to prepare residents to enter the community.

We stand at the crossroads. Disabled persons may find themselves once again segregated from the mainstream of educational, economic, and social life. On the other hand, this period of economic crisis may break down the old divisions between parents and professionals. In British Columbia, for example, where cutbacks have been severe, the social workers' association has adopted a social action perspective in opposing the government and has allied itself with the disabled and other minority groups. Such parent-professional-disabled person coalitions may lead to a further change in societal attitudes, and may secure support services for the future.

The place of traditional professionals at this time is unclear. Unless they assume an advocacy role and ally themselves with the movement to oppose reductions for families with a disabled member, however, they stand to re-create the antagonistic relationship between these families and professionals. Furthermore, they may be left to do "therapy" with families whose "problems" have been re-created by the social order.

IMPLICATIONS OF A SOCIAL ACTION PERSPECTIVE

The integration of a social action perspective into a family therapy framework can

- provide therapists with a clearer understanding of the social effects of disability on the family
- allow the therapist to join the family and create a therapeutic alliance by strategically punctuating the problem as "caused" by factors external to the family (The therapist's own conceptualization remains circular, however.)
- help family members to resist the paralyzing effects of stigmatization and take appropriate social action on their own behalf

Therapists cannot know the degree to which problems that appear in families with a disabled member result from the social experience of having a disabled member present. Certainly, these families are not immune to the problems faced by other families. However, to begin with problems that appear internal to the family is a strategic error. Such a focus further identifies the family as dysfunctional, generates "resistance" as the family struggles to avoid the therapist's definition of the problem, and risks increasing the family's self-blame, isolation, and withdrawal. A social action perspective avoids these pitfalls by defining difficulties experienced by the family with a disabled member as resulting primarily from the stigma and social barriers associated with disability. Inherent pathology within the family is not assumed. The therapist may intervene by

1. redefining the problem as one that occurs at the interface of the family and other systems
2. examining the family's belief system and challenging any identification with societal prejudice
3. introducing family members to information that allows them to put their experience into sociohistorical perspective
4. developing a perspective that anticipates and prepares for the future
5. aligning with the family in their efforts to secure better services and more equitable opportunities, and taking an advocacy role when necessary in representing the needs of the family to other professionals and systems

The adoption of a social action perspective has several implications for the training and practice of family therapy. Specifically, such a perspective calls for examining the work context and therapists' potential as social control agents, redefining therapists' relationship to these families, and developing a sociohistorical base.

Redefinition of the Problem

When the disabled and their families are referred for therapy, the identified problem is usually a particular person or relationship within the family. The first task of therapy is to redefine the problem at the level of the family and other systems in a manner that recognizes and legitimizes external pressures. This can empower family members to take concrete action to gain access to reference groups, support networks, and services within the community or to resolving conflicts between themselves and an outside system.

Redefinition may be difficult. Having been exposed to the many theories regarding their dysfunction, family members themselves may explain that their difficulties have internal causes. While validating their emotional experience, the therapist must connect their feelings to processes larger than the family. This parallels the therapy of gay and lesbian clients who may present the "causes" of their homosexuality or whose parents may blame themselves for their offspring's sexual orientation. Inquiries by either the therapist or client into internal causes reflect and reinforce the internalized societal prejudice (Martin, 1982).

Difficulties are also encountered if the therapist accepts the problem as defined by the referral source. In doing so, the therapist creates an implicit alliance with the referral source and may easily slip into the role of social control agent. To avoid this, the therapist must conceptualize the problem as a conflict between the referral source and the family. The therapist must then delicately intervene to help resolve the conflict and prevent escalation.

Examination of the Belief System

The degree to which members of a minority maintain self-esteem despite stigmatization depends on their ability to challenge their own internalized societal prejudice and identify with alternate values (Darling, 1979). Therapy may facilitate this process by making the connections between their distress and social conditions clear to the family and by challenging family beliefs that reflect the family's identification with the aggressor (in this case, the societal stigmatization of the disabled and their families). When successfully addressed in therapy, this identification is relinquished, and anger is directed against the source of oppression (Martin, 1982).

Introduction of Information

One way to make the connections between the family's distress and the social conditions explicit is to ask questions based on specific hypotheses (Selvini Palazzoli, Boscolo, Cecchin, & Prata, 1980). Within a social action paradigm, hypotheses generate information that allows family members to put their experience into a sociohistorical perspective. For example, questions to elicit information regarding the social context during the child's early years may include

- How was the family made aware of the child's disability?
- What experiences did family members have with professionals?
- What was the response of family members, extended family, and community?
- What difficulties were encountered in child care and education?
- What stresses were experienced by family members, and how did they respond?
- How did the child's birth change the lives and self-perception of family members?

The family's awareness of and response to changing social conditions may be explored through further questions:

- Who was most helpful and who was the most antagonistic to the family in the past and now?
- What did the parents believe was expected of disabled children and adults in the past? What is expected now?
- Who or what outside the family has most influenced family members? In what direction?
- What changes has the family seen in opportunities for the disabled member?
- Do family members believe such opportunities are increasing or decreasing?
- What do family members want in terms of opportunities?
- Have family members taken any action to bring about these opportunities?

Through the questioning process, the degree to which the family's problem is intricately interwoven into the social fabric begins to emerge. Some parents report great relief when the therapist acknowledges their struggles and their successes under difficult circumstances (Kratoville, 1975).

Development of Future Perspective

Families should be prepared in advance for difficult points of transition, such as school entrance, puberty, or leaving home. Problems may be presented by exploring issues with the family that will emerge in the future. In preparing the family for the child's leaving home, for example, key areas of exploration are the family's beliefs concerning the circumstances under which the disabled person will leave; its effect on the parents' relationship and their connection with the social network; the kinds of occupational, emotional, and sexual relationships the disabled person will form; living arrangements; financial security; and guardianship (Marlett, 1984). There are parallels in the constructs of next environment program planning (Brown, Hamre-Nietupski, Lyon, Branston, & Falvey, 1978). Rather than focusing intervention efforts on the current setting, teachers prepare the youngster and the family for the next least restrictive environment, thereby ensuring access to that environment and preparing families for the inevitability of change.

Actual alternatives depend on the social conditions that exist when the child reaches the particular transition point. Services gained in one era can be eroded in the next; solutions that worked for families in one era can become problems in the next. Therapists may ask questions concerning future services to introduce the idea that other services not considered may emerge. The very process of considering future alternatives prepares families for the risk and uncertainty in their futures. Both families and therapists must examine their solutions to problems in light of changing social conditions; they must remain aware of current influences through a connection with emerging social movements.

Alignment with the Family

As families become aware of the social roots of their difficulties, their emerging anger empowers them to adopt a social action perspective themselves. The therapist at this point aligns with the family, providing support and direction as family members reach out to other networks and subcultures, and begin to exert pressure to create the conditions for their optimal survival. The therapist needs a thorough knowledge of existing reference groups, services, and resources, as well as a sense of the most effective way for the family to approach the different organizations.

Because improved social opportunities and supports can be swept away by difficult economic times, the family may be the disabled person's only enduring and consistent support. The social action therapist validates the family as an ongoing resource for the disabled person, even while supporting the disabled young adult's capacity for making personal life decisions.

Examination of the Work Context

Social action therapists may encounter difficulties within their own work setting because they are often expected to function as agents of social control. For example, therapists may be expected to render families more cooperative and compliant with a social service agency's implicit norms. Conservative agencies are unlikely to support the therapist's taking an advocate role in representing the needs of the family to other professionals, community services, and government bodies.

To avoid triangulating families between social action therapists and conservative agencies, it may be necessary for agencies to change. The training of family therapists, however, rarely involves teaching skills for effecting change within agencies. Therapists in the field may find support by joining with other social action professionals to plan strategies and share common concerns, and by seeking further education on changing social service systems.

Redefinition of the Therapist-Family Relationship

When working within a social action perspective, the therapist becomes an advocate and collaborator with the family, rather than an authoritative expert. This is a strategic position to take with the disabled and their families, since they may reject a therapist who assumes a directive stance. In many current models of family therapy, however, the therapist assumes an expert position either directly or indirectly. The families' previous contact with professionals may also have prepared them to cast therapists into this role.

Ways must be found, therefore, not only for therapists to remove themselves from this role, but also to make it clear to the family that they have done so. For example, therapists may discuss the family's reluctance to trust and explore with family members their past experiences with professionals. The questioning process communicates to the family the "differentness" of this therapist and shows how problems have evolved, in part, through their interaction with professionals. The therapist offers to the family a relationship based on collaboration, acknowledging both the therapist's expertise in human processes and the family's expertise in living with a disabled person.

Development of a Sociohistorical Base

Training for therapists must focus on social and political issues relating to disability. Therapists require a sociohistorical base in order to understand the particular family in therapy in terms of the changing social forces on the family as the child matures. In order to confront and deal with the therapists' own culturally ingrained responses to disability, it is also desirable for training programs to include contact with disabled persons and activists.

CONCLUSION

The final implications of adopting a social action perspective in therapy with families that have a disabled member are unknown. If this perspective is adopted by a large number of family therapists in their work with the disabled, the same lens may be applied to work with other minority groups and, eventually, to all families in therapy. The ultimate impact on family therapy is unpredictable, but it may call into question some of our most basic assumptions.

REFERENCES

Bishop, D., & Epstein, N. (1980). Family problems and disability. In D. Bishop (Ed.), *Behavioral problems and the disabled*. Baltimore: Williams & Wilkins.

Bowe, F. (1978). *Handicapping America*. New York: Harper & Row.

Brown, L., Hamre-Nietupski, S., Lyon, S., Branston, M., & Falvey, M. (1978). Curricular strategies for developing longitudinal interactions between severely handicapped students and others and curricular strategies for teaching severely handicapped students to acquire and perform skills in response to naturally-occurring cues and correction procedures. Vol. 8, Part 1. Madison, Wisc.: Madison Metropolitan School District.

Darling, R. (1979). *Families against society: A study of reactions to children with birth defects*. Beverly Hills, CA: Sage.

Ferrari, M., Mathews, W., & Barabas, (1983). The family and the child with epilepsy. *Family Process, 22*(1), 53–59.

Flanigan, P. (1970). *Orientation to mental retardation*. Toronto: National Institute of Mental Retardation.

Gliedman, J., & Roth, W. (1980). *The unexpected minority*. New York: Harcourt Brace Jovanovich.

Heumann, J. (1979). Handicap and disability. In J. Hourihin (Ed.), *Disability: Our challenge.* New York: Teachers College, Columbia University.

Hourihin, J. (Ed.). (1979). *Disability: Our challenge.* New York: Teachers College, Columbia University.

James, K., & McIntyre, D. (1983). The reproduction of mothering: The social role of family therapy? *Journal of Marital and Family Therapy, 9*(2), 119–129.

Kanner, L. (1964). *A history of the care and study of the mentally retarded.* Springfield, IL: Charles C Thomas.

Kaslow, F., & Cooper, B. (1978). Family therapy with the learning disabled child and his/her family. *Journal of Marriage and Family Therapy, 4*(1), 41–49.

Kratoville, M. (1975). What parents need to hear. In L. Buscaglia (Ed.), *The disabled and their parents: A counselling challenge.* Thorofare, Nova Scotia: Charles Slack.

Kugel, R., & Wolfensberger, W. (1969). *Changing patterns in residential services for the mentally retarded.* Washington, DC: President's Committee on Mental Retardation.

Leob, R. (1977). Group therapy for parents of mentally retarded children. *Journal of Marriage and Family Counseling, 3*(2), 77–83.

Marlett, N.J. (1978). Normalization, socialization and integration. In J.P. Das & D. Baine (Eds.), *Mental retardation for special educators.* Springfield, IL: Charles C Thomas.

Marlett, N.J. (1984). Determination of personal competence: Important considerations for parents, service providers, and professionals. In A. Appolini, & N. Vincent (Eds.), *Guardianship, lifelong protection for persons with developmental disabilities.* Baltimore: Paul H. Brookes.

Martin, A. (1982). Some issues in the treatment of gay and lesbian clients. *Psychotherapy: Theory, Research and Practice, 19*(3), 341–348.

Palazzoli, Selvini M., Boscolo, L., Cecchin, G., & Prata, G. (1980). Hypothesizing-circulants-neutrality: Three guidelines for the conductor of the session. *Family Process, 19*(1), 3–12.

Philp, M., & Duckworth, D. (1982). *Children with disabilities and their families: A review of research.* Windsor, England: Nelson Publishing Co.

Rule, J. (1971). The problem with social problems. *Politics and Society, 2*(1), 47–56.

Shapiro, R., & Harris, R. (1976). Family therapy in treatment of the deaf: A case report. *Family Process, 15*(1), 83–96.

Turner, A. (1980). Therapy with families of a mentally retarded child. *Journal of Marriage and Family Therapy, 6*(2), 167–170.

Woodard, L., & Woodard, B. (1982). A case of the blind leading the "blind": Reframing a physical handicap as competence. *Family Process, 21*(3), 291–294.

10. Social Network Interventions for Families That Have a Handicapped Child

Michael Berger

This paper is dedicated to William A. Bricker, in memoriam.

Acknowledgments: The comments of Martha Foster, Ph.D., Debbie Daniels-Mohring, Jim Kochalka, and C. Wayne Jones on previous drafts of the paper are gratefully appreciated.

WORKING WITH A FAMILY THAT HAS A HANDICAPPED CHILD IS SIMILAR to working with any family that has a child-related problem in the kinds of information collected, the structural and strategic tactics used (Fisch, Weakland, & Segal, 1982; Haley, 1976; Minuchin & Fishman, 1981), and the concepts that characterize successful ways of changing families. There are additional circumstances and nuances that should be considered when working with a family with a handicapped child, however.

These families are likely to be intensely involved with a number of different service systems (Darling, 1979; Gorham, Des Jardins, Page, Pettis, & Scheiber, 1975). While many families possess the resources required to deal with a particular child problem, provided that their current way of dealing with the problem is altered (Fisch et al., 1982; Haley, 1976; Minuchin, 1974), few families with a severely or multiply handicapped child have the resources necessary to provide the training, equipment, and care that such a child needs in order to develop as normally as possible. Thus, in order to support the growth of their handicapped child, these families must deal with a number of service systems, often on an ongoing basis, each of which focuses on a different aspect of the child's problem (Gorham et al., 1975; Schwartz, 1970). Frequently, these services are organized in such a way that it is difficult for a family to coordinate them.

The mother usually arranges for the youngster's treatment. Thus, in families with a handicapped child, there is often a close mother-child dyad. This closeness is intensified by the fact that many agencies present their treatment programs to parents as if they *must* be carried out, even at the expense of other aspects of family life (Foster, Berger, & McLean, 1981). In order to obtain services, families may feel obliged to comply with agency demands. The responsibility for carrying out these treatments is usually placed on the mother, who, therefore, legitimately worries that she is neglecting the handicapped child if she focuses on her other children, her marriage, or herself.

Another common problem is the tendency for family members to arrange their lives around the handicapping condition as if it were the central fact about the family. When rigid and persistent, such patterns of organization often become detrimental to family members, preventing them from growing and changing in response to their own needs (Berger, 1984; Darling, 1979; Foster & Berger, 1979).

Social network interventions can be used to help families with handicapped children. The social network includes the persons important to family members, such as extended family members, friends, neighbors, and professionals involved with the handicapped child or with other family members. Given the importance of service systems to families with handicapped children and the importance of extended family and friends to most families, it is crucial for the social network to be the therapist's unit of conceptualization. The particular unit directly treated in any given instance should be determined by pragmatic considerations; any unit that allows the therapist to help the family deal with its problems is a reasonable one (Berger & Jurkovic, 1984; Dammann & Berger, 1983; Scheflen, 1980).

INTERVENTIONS TO PRESERVE NETWORK INTEGRITY

Following the diagnosis of a handicapping condition in a child, families are likely to reduce their contact with neighbors, friends, and extended family members (Darling, 1979; Farber, 1968; Holt, 1958). A temporary reduction in contact with social network members may be useful in that it permits family members to deal with the handicapping condition before they share this new fact with others. In extreme cases, however, the family ceases to deal with persons who are not directly connected to the handicapped child, limiting contact to service providers and other parents of handicapped children. In order to prevent such extreme restrictions, the therapist should work with the family and its social network, keeping the family in contact with its network members and helping both the family and the network deal with the presence of a handicapped child in the family.

This can be done in a variety of ways. The therapist may coach the parents in ways to maintain their ties to network members while they find out what the handicapped child needs and what changes in the family and network will be required in order to meet these new demands (Bowen, 1976; Hollister, 1978). The therapist may meet directly with the family and the network, helping them to share their concerns about the handicapped child and about the effects of the handicapping condition on the family and the network (Berger, 1984; Berger & Fowlkes, 1980). Such meetings usually have both a ritual and a problem-solving function. The mere facts that the meetings are held, that network members do attend, and that network members survive the anticipated difficulties of talking about the handicapped child powerfully communicate to family and network members that they are important to one another and that the network has the resources to deal with the problems it confronts. Such meetings can also be used to construct solutions to child-rearing problems, for example, to work out a plan for several family or network members to share the tasks of obtaining services or of training the handicapped child so that these tasks do not fall solely on the child's mother. Berger (1984) described one such network intervention in detail.

The therapist may meet first with the parents and then with the parents and parts of the network (Dammann & Berger, 1983).

Case Example: Across the Generations

I first met with the Howards after their 10-year-old son, Michael, had been tested and found to have significant learning disabilities. Michael had been a difficult child since birth. Although Mrs. Howard had long felt that Michael had neurological or learning disabilities, no one in the extended family had agreed with her. Thus, she had been feeling incompetent about her parenting of Michael for years. At the time of the first meeting, Mr. and Mrs. Howard expressed concern about Michael's behavior problems in school and at home with his younger sister, his temper tantrums, and his "lack of self-esteem." In addition, the Howards were interested in reorganizing the family so as to help Michael do as well in school as possible.

In the first interview, I obtained a developmental history and a history of the parents' involvement with Michael's difficulties. I also obtained a multigenerational history on each parent. Mrs. Howard was the elder of two children. She had been her father's darling, but she had been in conflict with her mother since adolescence. At present, this conflict centered around Michael; Mrs. Howard's mother thought she could be much more successful in dealing with Michael. Mr. Howard's parents had divorced. He had spent his adolescence living with his mother; his stepfather, a retired career serviceman; and his younger brother. He had distanced himself from his family in adolescence, and that distance was still maintained, although he had some contact with his mother. At the time of therapy, Mrs. Howard served as the go-between between Mr. Howard and his mother and stepfather.

Two things became clear in this interview. Both sets of grandparents were very involved with Michael, and Mrs. Howard felt that she would not be supported in dealing with Michael. After working out some new daily routines at home and some changes in the ways that teachers dealt with Michael at school so that the Howards were feeling some success in dealing with Michael, I asked to meet with both sets of grandparents. The Howards said they were willing to do this, but they preferred for me to meet separately with each set of grandparents, since "Mrs. Howard's parents will do all the talking, and you won't get anything out of Mr. Howard's parents unless you see them separately."

I scheduled a meeting first with the Howards and the maternal grandparents. After describing Michael's learning disabilities and the ways in which they had made it necessary to restructure his home environment, I indicated the changes that his parents had already made, explained that Michael needed consistent structure in his environment, and stressed how important it was that his grandparents adopt the new ways of dealing with him. The grandparents agreed to this.

I then asked Mrs. Howard's mother whether she had been surprised to learn that Michael had learning disabilities. This led her into a discussion of her past worries about Michael, which led, in turn, to a quite moving discussion of her worries about Mrs. Howard when she was a child. Since Mrs. Howard had been feeling that she was a failure with Michael, I suggested that it was likely to take her some time to notice how well she had been doing with him. The grandmother agreed, and I asked whether she would help her daughter by convincing her that she was doing a good job with Michael. In response to this, Mrs. Howard reiterated her belief that her mother thought she was failing with Michael, while the grandmother described her pain about feeling that not only had she been unable to parent her daughter successfully, but also she had been unable to help her daughter parent Michael.

Noting that both the parents and the grandparents were concerned about Michael's lack of self-esteem, I said that I thought Michael felt bad about himself because he had been failing in school for several years, even though this was through no fault of his own. Things were beginning to go better for him at school, I continued, but I thought it would take some time before he noticed this and even more time before he changed his unfortunately low view of himself. Everyone agreed, so I then wondered whether Mrs. Howard, who had held an unfortunately low view of her parenting of Michael for several years now, might be going through a similar process. The grandparents agreed that such might be the case. Remarking on Mrs. Howard's closeness to her father, I asked him if he would help his wife help his daughter by telling her that she was doing well with Michael. He agreed to do this, and the grandmother agreed to let him, although she protested that she had already told her daughter this. I agreed, but suggested that she might have to do it several times before her daughter changed the way she thought about herself.

The initial difficulty in getting the paternal grandparents to collaborate with the parents was the stepfather's feeling that there would have been no problems with Michael if Mr. Howard had not "let his wife work." While this disagreement was not resolved in the session, the parents were able to make it clear that they both wanted Mrs. Howard to work and they both felt that her working was not detrimental to Michael. In addition, the grandparents agreed to put aside these differences and to adopt the new ways of dealing with Michael; the new ways seemed stricter, which pleased the stepfather. In a subsequent discussion with the parents, I framed the disagreement as a normal problem between couples and their in-laws. The couple accepted this reframing and began work on setting boundaries with both sets of parents.

The meetings with the parents and grandparents, then, kept the participants in contact with one another as they negotiated a new definition of Michael's problem and what to do about it. The new frame that was developed during these meetings—differences between couples and their in-laws are normal and predictable events—underplayed the centrality of Michael's handicap to the family and the network.

In summary, in order to maintain network integrity the therapist must help create a ritual that allows network members to accept the fact of the child's handicapping condition while still maintaining ties to family members that do not define them mainly as "the family of a handicapped child" (Berger, 1984; Dammann & Berger, 1983).

FAMILY PROBLEM SOLVING

Clinicians have most commonly used social network meetings as a means to solve family problems (Attneave, 1976). To accomplish this, the therapist meets with the units of the family network that have the resources necessary to solve the problems. Network interventions of a therapist include meeting with the professionals in a family's network to coordinate their efforts for the family when such efforts have previously been fragmented or have pushed family members in contradictory directions (Hoffman & Long, 1969) or meeting with all the people involved with the handicapped child to work out a consistent child care schedule and set of routines.

It is often necessary to negotiate a common definition of the situation, a common framing of the problem, in order to coordinate action. In this instance, the therapist helps network members construct a definition of the situation that is acceptable to all of them so that they will collaborate (Minuchin & Fishman, 1981). The therapist must first block off certain definitions of the situation in order to increase the likelihood that other definitions will be chosen.

Case Example: Fallen through the Cracks

> Recently, I attended an education planning meeting about a 17-year-old girl who suffers from a genetic condition that results in mental retardation, obesity, and blindness. In addition, because she had struck her

mother (she is quite a large girl) and used foul language at her father, she had been hospitalized for several weeks at a psychiatric hospital several summers ago. For the past 2 years, she had attended a residential school for the blind, spending summers with her mother. (Her parents were divorced, but maintained almost constant contact with one another because of their daughter.) The meeting had been called because the girl had not done well academically and had not been behaving well at the school for the blind. School personnel felt that her difficulties were caused by her "emotional disturbance," a diagnosis based on her previous psychiatric hospitalization, while her parents felt that the school did not provide their daughter with either sufficient environmental structure or sufficient vocational instruction.

The purpose of the meeting was to devise a treatment plan for the girl for the coming year. The meeting began with a statement from the representative of the school for the blind that the school would no longer accept the girl. The father said that he also thought the school was an inappropriate placement and asked whether the local school system would work out a more suitable placement. The chairperson indicated that the school system had no other placement to offer and asked me for my opinion. I said that the most appropriate program would combine vocational training with training in self-help skills with the ultimate goal of helping the girl leave home to live independently. The chairperson said that the school system could not provide vocational training, that only the training center could do that. In turn, the representative of the training center said that, legally, the school system had to serve the girl and that, in addition, the girl would require training that was not available at the training center to overcome her visual impairment.

Although the school system and the training center had never worked out a joint program, the girl's mother made a moving speech about how her daughter had always fallen between the cracks in service systems and pleaded for a collaborative program. The representative of the school for the blind said the girl was "too emotionally disturbed to function successfully in such a program." When asked whether I agreed with that assessment, I responded not only that the girl had no psychiatric condition, but also that, given appropriate structure, the girl did not engage in the behaviors that disturbed the school or had resulted in her previous hospitalization. The mother corroborated this and noted that, since she and her ex-husband had been working together, there had not been a need to hospitalize the girl. The chairperson reiterated that no joint program could be worked out if the girl had an emotional problem. After several repetitions of parts of the above sequence, the meeting was adjourned. Within a week, the school system and training center had worked out a joint program.

This outcome came about, in part, because the special education and training center representatives were moved by the parents' plight. They were also excited about the opportunity to do something that would be innovative and would make a difference in this girl's life. Defining the girl as someone who would easily benefit from clear structure and appropriate services was reinforcing to the agencies who worked with her. In order to have this definition prevail, it was necessary to keep school and training center personnel from labeling the girl as emotionally disturbed.

It is common for the therapist in such meetings to play a role that is somewhere between that of an arbitrator in a labor dispute and that of an advocate for the child and family. As an arbitrator, the task is to develop a definition of the situation that enables the participants to work together for the benefit of the client (Hobbs, 1982). As an advocate, the task is to make sure that the interests of the child and family are not sacrificed to the procedures of service agencies. As the father of the girl in the previous example said to me after the meeting: "You know, they wouldn't have listened to me if I had said what you did. But they *would* listen to a doctor." I said I was sorry to have to agree that he was correct but I was also glad that he had been smart enough to "take me into the meeting as his hired gun." He nodded, wearily.

NETWORK MEETINGS AS A CONTEXT FOR ENACTMENTS

While all the therapist's usual techniques (e.g., joining, reframing, tracking sequences, mapping, and changing organizational structures) are relevant to the conduct of effective network interventions, these interventions are a particularly good context for the use of enactments. Network members know one another well and have been important to one another over long periods of time. If the therapist can help create a context in which network members act differently with one another, that new behavior will reverberate through the numerous transactions that network members have with each other. Network interventions, then, are especially powerful contexts for the use of enactments that alter network members' definition of the handicapping condition or of what needs to be done about that condition.

Case Example: Climbing the Mountain

After the joint program was developed between the school system and the training center, the girl and her family were told that, if she did well in the program during the summer, she would be placed in a vocational training program at the center during the fall. In addition, work would be done to prepare her to function successfully in a half-way house. To increase the girl's chance of succeeding in the summer program, the parents hired two graduate students to work with the girl individually on self-control and self-care tasks.

The girl did well in all the training situations during the summer. It was clear to the students, however, that both the center staff and the girl's parents were hesitant to believe that she was doing as well as she was and that she would continue to do well. A week before the meeting to assess the girl's achievements during the summer, the students told me that the girl had climbed down a local mountain all by herself the previous weekend. This was a considerable achievement for the girl, for a blind person, and for anyone not skilled in mountaineering. Impressed by the girl's accomplishment, the students devised an enactment to be used during the assessment meeting.

At the meeting, all the parties involved except the girl (i.e., her parents, the students, the workers from the center) reviewed their work during the summer. All agreed that the girl had done well, but there was some concern about her ability to continue to do well, particularly since she would be more independent. At this point, one of the students asked if the girl could enter the room, since she had "something important to tell the group." The group consented; the girl told the story of climbing down the mountain. Her parents cried while listening to the story, and the staff were also visibly impressed. The enactment proved successful, and the girl was admitted to the vocational training program.

ENGAGING NETWORK MEMBERS IN TREATMENT

A variety of strategies can be used to get network members to participate in network meetings. Therapists who direct the setting in which they function can mandate participation in network meetings. (Interestingly, when I directed a setting and could do this, less than 2% of families questioned the necessity of these meetings [Berger, 1984; Berger & Fowlkes, 1980].) A more step-by-step approach is to begin working with nuclear family members, develop a relationship with them, and then demonstrate the need for the involvement of extended family members or friends (Berger & Daniels-Mohring, 1982; Dammann & Berger, 1983). The strategy most likely to work with the professionals who are part of the family's social network is to ask for a meeting to coordinate the activity of all the professionals involved with the family. This strategy, as Todd (1984) noted, is most likely to work when the family therapist is viewed, not as seeking control over the case, but as being willing to do the time-consuming work of case coordination as a favor to his or her professional colleagues. (For other descriptions of ways to engage people in network interventions, see Attneave, 1976, and Speck & Attneave, 1973.)

CONCLUSION

A number of writers have argued recently that a more ecological assessment of the context of a family is needed (Berger & Jurkovic, 1984; Coppersmith, 1983; Keeney, 1983; Scheflen, 1980). Such an assessment should include individuals, subsystems within the family, the family as a whole, the social network, and the community. An ecological approach is essential with regard to families with handicapped children, since the fate of these families is so intertwined with the kinds of support they receive from personal and service networks (Darling, 1979; Gorham et al., 1975). Therapists who work with such families, therefore, must learn to intervene in such a way as to be helpful both to the families and to the other elements of this larger context.

REFERENCES

Attneave, C. (1976). Social networks as the unit of intervention. In P. Guerin (Ed.), *Family therapy: Theory and practice*. New York: Gardner.

Berger, M. (1984). Systems therapy and special education settings. In M. Berger & G. Jurkovic (Eds.), *Family therapy in context: The practice of systemic therapy in community settings*. San Francisco: Jossey-Bass.

Berger, M., & Daniels-Mohring, D. (1982). The strategic use of "Bowenian" formulations. *Journal of Strategic and Systemic Therapies, 1,* 50–56.

Berger, M., & Fowlkes, M. (1980). The family intervention project: A family network model for serving young handicapped children. *Young Children, 35,* 22–32.

Berger, M., & Jurkovic, G. (Eds.). (1984). *Family therapy in context: The practice of systemic therapy in community settings*. San Francisco: Jossey-Bass.

Bowen, M. (1976). Family reaction to death. In P. Guerin (Ed.), *Family therapy: Theory and practice*. New York: Gardner.

Coppersmith, E.I. (1983). The family and public service systems: An assessment method. In B. Keeney (Ed.), *Diagnosis and assessment in family therapy*. Rockville, MD: Aspen Systems Corporation.

Dammann, C., & Berger, M. (1983). Household and family: Creating a viable treatment unit. *Journal of Strategic and Systemic Therapies, 2*(3), 67–73.

Darling, R. (1979). *Families against society*. New York: Russell Sage.

Farber, B. (1968). *Mental retardation: Its social context and social consequences*. Boston: Houghton Mifflin.

Fisch, R., Weakland, J., & Segal, L. (1982). *The tactics of change: Doing therapy briefly.* San Francisco: Jossey-Bass.

Foster, M., & Berger, M. (1979). Structural family therapy: Applications in programs for preschool handicapped children. *Journal of the Division of Early Childhood, 1,* 52–58.

Foster, M., Berger, M., & McLean, M. (1981). Rethinking a good idea: A reassessment of parent involvement. *Topics in Early Childhood Special Education, 1,* 55–65.

Gorham, K., Des Jardins, C., Page, R., Pettis, E., & Scheiber, B. (1975). Effect on parents. In N. Hobbs (Ed.), *Issues in the classification of children* (Vol. 2). San Francisco: Jossey-Bass.

Haley, J. (1976). *Problem-solving therapy.* San Francisco: Jossey-Bass.

Hobbs, N. (1982). *The troubled and the troubling child.* San Francisco: Jossey-Bass.

Hoffman, L., & Long, L. (1969). A systems dilemma. *Family Process, 8,* 211–234.

Hollister, M. (1978). Families who experience the death of a child. In R. Sagar (Ed.), *Georgetown Family Symposia* (Vol. 3). Washington, DC: Georgetown University Family Studies Center.

Holt, M. (1958). Home care of severely retarded children. *Pediatrics, 22,* 744–754.

Keeney, B. (Ed.). (1983). *Diagnosis and assessment in family therapy.* Rockville, MD: Aspen Systems Corporation.

Minuchin, S. (1974). *Families and family therapy.* Cambridge: Harvard University Press.

Minuchin, S., & Fishman, C. (1981). *Techniques of family therapy.* Cambridge: Harvard University Press.

Scheflen, A. (1980). *Levels of schizophrenia.* New York: Brunner/Mazel.

Schwartz, C. (1970). Strategies and tactics of mothers of mentally retarded children for dealing with the medical care system. In N. Bernstein (Ed.), *Diminished people.* Boston: Little, Brown.

Speck, R., & Attneave, A. (1973). *Family networks.* New York: Pantheon.

Todd, T. (1984). Administrative issues and family systems therapy: What happens when a family therapist is granted his or her wish for power. In M. Berger & G. Jurkovic (Eds.), *Family therapy in context: The practice of systemic therapy in community settings.* San Francisco: Jossey-Bass.

11. Retarded Adults, Their Families, and Larger Systems: A New Role for the Family Therapist

Stephen Bloomfield
Scott Nielsen
Lauren Kaplan

Donna, a 22-year-old, moderately retarded woman had lived in a supervised apartment for about a year. Her parents, in their mid-60s, had placed Donna there, as they did "not know how long we have left." The residential staff reported that Donna had been behaving in a progressively violent manner and had been showing psychotic symptoms.

The parents thought the staff was "too young to really understand Donna." The staff thought, in the words of one staff member, that the couple was "detouring their covert conflicts through Donna." Although the case manager empathized with both parties, she became increasingly frustrated in trying to find a workable solution and called in a family therapy consultant. The case manager thought the client, her parents, and the service providers were all contributing to the conflicts, and she hoped family therapy would resolve the difficulties.

THIS SITUATION IS NOT UNUSUAL WHEN A MENTALLY RETARDED ADULT is involved. The problem is complex, as it involves the intersecting dynamics of at least two systems with notably different purposes: the family and various service providers. Furthermore, these types of conflicts occur within the semipublic context of helping institutions, and the success of one system could easily be seen as the failure of the others.

The problem addressed in this paper is threefold. First, the presenting population, mentally retarded adults, is one that is generally unfamiliar to family and other therapists. Second, the developmental issues experienced by families with a retarded adult member are different from and often more complex than the norm. Third, but most central, is the problematic interaction between a family and the social service systems that are designed to help them.

The systemic family therapist can adopt a new role in working with systems organized around a mentally retarded adult. The way of working may not look like therapy; indeed, at times, recommends ignoring therapy. The task of the family therapist in working with retarded adults, their families, and larger systems is to develop a method of intervention that avoids blaming anyone and allows the system to change. The method outlined here frees the family therapist from hierarchical struggles with other professionals. It is contrary to the concept that family therapy is the only appropriate treatment modality. Instead, it allows psychotherapists a chance to provide psychotherapy, case managers a chance to manage, advocacy groups a chance to advocate, and behavioral managers a chance to manage behavior.

THE PROBLEM

Therapy and the Mentally Retarded

Until recently, therapists have found retarded adults a difficult population to serve. Traditionally, the professional services provided have been in the areas of educational or vocational training (Turner, 1980). Supplemented by advocacy, case management, and behavioral management programs, treatment has been either long-term institutionalization or the provision of services focused on normalization (Wolfensberger, 1972). One reason for this has been that psychotherapists, family therapists included, have been neither willing nor able to provide services to mentally retarded people. Therapists have viewed the problems of the retarded as impossible to ameliorate therapeutically. Therapists' lack of experience with the population and the belief that the problems of the retarded are dominated by their biological condition have been offered as the reasons that therapy is not a useful solution. Furthermore, some advocacy groups have suggested that therapy is not normal, which also allows professionals to deny needed services. Injunctions against therapy are ill-founded, however. Retarded people and their families are subject to the same difficulties and problems encountered by anyone. If any person needs or is entitled to use therapy, so do they.

Developmental Issues

The developmental issues in families with retarded children have both normative and unique qualities. As most young people leave their parental homes, they become more fully responsible for organizing and supervising their own financial and emotional support (Carter & McGoldrick, 1980). When retarded adult children leave home, they, too, are expected to show more independent living skills. The most critical aspect of this change, however, is the transition from the daily supervision of one set of caregivers—parents—to that of another—staff of a residential program. Many parents experience ambivalence about their young adult children moving out on their own; and the need for continued supervision makes the parents of the retarded particularly susceptible to worry. Additionally, the placement of a retarded adult child is often complicated by the fact that parents are aging and approaching death. A frequent factor in the placement decision is the growing urgency of the question "What happens to our child after we are gone?" The management of one major developmental transition is work enough for most families, but the confluence of two complex developmental events—leaving home and parental mortality—is certainly enough to encourage unusual behavior from one or more family members.

Larger Systems Issues

It is important and possible to provide therapy to families with a retarded member just as therapy would be provided for any family and yet understand the uniqueness of the developmental issues that these families face on an individual, familial, and societal levels. The critical issue in resolving conflicts that arise in these types of situations has to do with the interaction between the client/family system and the service system, however. It is not only the clients or their families that need to change, but the network of service systems organized around them that should be considered the unit of treatment.

Families with a retarded adult member have often been involved with professional helpers for years. By virtue of that involvement alone, these families qualify to be called "multiproblem" families, as such families in the literature are labeled not by the multitude and persistence of their problems, but by the multitude and persistence of their agency contacts. The multiproblem label is merely blameful of families. It is more useful and exact to distinguish between families that are agency-engaged and those that are agency-enmeshed. Certainly, many families with a retarded child can be agency-engaged for many years by participating in treatment planning, utilizing services, and negotiating conflicts with providers, all without a family member demonstrating increasingly dysfunctional behavior. In a number of cases, however, one symptom or conflict follows another, policy-altering efforts have no impact, and agencies connect through family crises rather than planned service coordination, all of which render families more involved with the agencies that are designed to help them reduce their problems. Families in these cases, which consume the most effort with the least results and in which nobody and everybody seems to be to blame, can be referred to as agency-enmeshed. For some reason, these families have lost their capacity to steer their own course of development, and neither they nor the agencies appear capable of helping them regain their relative autonomy.

Systemic family therapy has proved a successful paradigm in the assessment of and intervention with dysfunctional family systems. The shift from an individual perspective to a family perspective demands a second shift, which is now occurring in the field. The focus on the family as a whole is changing to include the family's interaction with other systems in a larger social context. Family therapists have always seen environmental factors as important, but they have generally focused on the family as the unit of treatment. For example, Minuchin (1974), identified four stressors that affect a family's ability to adapt within its environment: (1) the stressful contact of one member with extrafamilial forces, (2) the stressful contact of the whole family with extrafamilial forces, (3) stress around a family life cycle transition, and (4) stress around idiosyncratic problems. As discussed previously, the leaving home crisis that this family faced satisfies stressors (3) and (4), as a life cycle event that has unique qualities. Clearly, a family with a retarded adult member can easily experience all four stressors. Minuchin implied that, if one stressor can contribute to dysfunction, the experience of all four can be overwhelming.

Given these stressors, it is not just the family system that must change when a conflict arises. Systemic family therapy theory and its techniques can be applied to make changes in systems larger than, yet inclusive of, a dysfunctional family or member. It is this larger context of interacting family and service systems that is seen as the unit of treatment in resolving the agency enmeshment of families with a retarded adult member. Ecological thinkers (Aponte, 1981) have proposed that a family system is best defined in relation to the other systems with which the family interacts. Goolishan and Anderson (1981) suggested that, in order to be successful, the therapist must include people outside the family in formulations and treatment. Haley (1980) suggested that the therapist must be completely in charge of the direction of treatment, somehow gaining control of the other helpers involved. These suggestions are useful in that they begin to expand the family therapist's frame of reference.

Selvini Palazzoli, Boscolo, Cecchin, and Prata (1980) dealt most insightfully with the problem of the referring person. They felt that part of the assessment must include the nature and functioning of the person making the referral as this is a key to understanding a problematic interaction that the family is experiencing. Based on this understanding, therapists are then free to include, exclude, or ignore this person.

Coppersmith (1983) broadened these formulations by suggesting that families may provide a homeostatic mechanism for the interaction of two or more larger systems. For example, the family that seems "resistant" to therapy at one mental health center may simply be loyal to a caseworker at another agency. This "resistance" becomes one means of maintaining the relationship between the two agencies. Coppersmith cautioned therapists about assuming where the problem lies, however:

Working within the boundaries of the family, when the correct level for intervention is either at the interface of the family and larger systems, or within larger systems, may place the family therapist in the paradoxical position of supporting stress by the very actions intended to relieve stress.

The critical larger system interface is characterized by conflict and competition between service providers and families as all parties work in the "best interest" of the retarded adult. Sometimes, service providers compete among themselves, while parents watch with growing frustration. Most often, however, parents join the fray. The parties end up in a symmetrical escalation that no one wants nor understands how to stop. Since they cannot give up and their efforts seem to intensify the problem, someone in the network calls for additional help. This extra help either adds to the confusion and the cycle continues on as it did before, or it creates a new perspective on the problem and offers the group a way to work in a more complementary fashion.

The question remains, if the family-larger system interface is the appropriate level for intervention, how does the therapist work?

Donna, the patient discussed earlier, had been living at home with her parents since birth, except for a 2-year placement in an out-of-state educational residential facility. Her father, Mr. Perlman, was a private construction contractor in his mid-60s; her mother was an antique dealer in her early 60s. At the time of the consultation, Donna had been living in a supervised apartment for approximately 1 year and was involved in a day vocation program. A psychiatrist employed by the residential program was providing psychotherapeutic services and monitoring her medication.

The consultant's primary contact was with the case manager assigned to work with Donna. Her role was complicated, as it consisted of coordinating a range of services for Donna, monitoring these services, and advocating for Donna's best interest. The decision to utilize a family therapy consultant was based on what was described as Donna's problematic behavior. She was described as behaving progressively more violently and as manifesting psychotic symptoms. To assess the problem and determine the most useful level of intervention, the consultant met with the residential staff at the apartment, Donna's parents in their home, and the case manager at her office.

The residential staff were committed to a policy of normalization and were offended that Mr. Perlman would hold a door for Donna when she entered a room. They felt this was patronizing and kept Donna in a child-like role. The staff reported that Donna would call out her father's name when she showered. One policy prohibited visits from parents in the first 6 months, but the parents were reported to have visited the apartment unannounced. Furthermore, they visited a weekend staff member at her other job in order to persuade her to work more closely with Donna. The residential staff thought that the parents were overinvolved with Donna and interfered with their treatment program. It was thought that the couple were, in the words of one staff member, "detouring their covert conflicts through Donna." The staff expressed sentiments that the Perlmans were in need of couples therapy.

The parents expressed feelings of guilt regarding what they viewed as their abandonment of Donna. They felt that for 21 years they had been able to care for her, but "now that we don't know how long we have left" they felt that they had to institutionalize her. They did not trust the residential staff, however. Mr. Perlman did not understand the staff's attitude regarding his holding the door for Donna. He told the consultant, "After all, I hold the door for my wife." When asked about visiting the relief staff person at her other job, the Perlmans reported the same events as the staff. They stated that they did so because they thought the woman, who was older than the regular staff, could better relate to Donna. They thought the residential staff "were too young to really understand Donna." Mr. and Mrs. Perlman also expressed concern that Donna was receiving psychotropic medication and thought the drugs were not necessary.

The consultant's meeting with the case manager confirmed the earlier reports. There was no argument about the facts. The case manager expressed frustration, since she received twice weekly calls from the parents and from their lawyer advocate. She received almost daily calls from the residential staff, who threatened to terminate services if the parents did not leave Donna alone. The case manager stated that she understood and empathized with both the residential staff and parents.

Consultant's Hypothesis and Prescriptions

The consultant viewed each of the three parties as similarly concerned about Donna's welfare, although each from different perspectives. The familial and professional orientations to Donna's care differed in their goals. Also, the parents did not belong to the same generation as most of the service providers. Each party operated as if they were "a set of parents," however. The consultant's hypothesis after these three meetings was that Donna's two or three "sets of parents" were in conflict and were vying for Donna's loyalty. Donna was attempting to remain loyal to all, even at her own expense. She was, furthermore, trying to bring them together and to diffuse the conflict as she acted mad or bad.

Two meetings with the residential staff, the parents, Donna, and the case manager were convened in order to gather interactional information regarding the various subsystems and to observe Donna in a safe forum with her different "sets of parents." The first session was a problem-focused initial interview. At the conclusion of this session, the consultant held a meeting with the case manager to explain the hypothesis and develop a strategy for the next session.

The second session was convened by the case manager and was to be the final session. One purpose of the second meeting was to disengage the consultant and establish the case manager as the outside expert. The strategy was to develop a subsystem to decide the future course of treatment based upon coordination rather than competition for control of the case. It was not expected that establishing complementary and clearly defined roles could be effected with a direct problem-solving approach and so techniques common to systemic family therapy were used. The session had two parts, one in which the consultant provided information that framed the situation in a changeable manner and the second in which the parties worked together to make specific decisions.

The session opened with a report to the group, including recommendations. The recommendations positively connoted everyone's behavior as demonstrating overwhelming concern for Donna's well-being, and Donna's behavior as her only, however misguided, way of bringing these caregivers together. The discussion made clear that she no longer needed to do this, since these adults could really handle it themselves. The complementarity that could exist between the parents, who had known and cared for Donna for twenty-one years, and the staff, who were closer to her own age, was explained. A useful developmental framing was developed, describing this situation as similar to that of a young adult going off to college. The necessity of forming new relationships and establishing a new household was discussed in that context. Residential staff were asked to remember what it was like for them, and how they felt about all the difficulties inherent in becoming independent. It was suggested that in that process people retain a place in their parent's home although they have their own home and that parents are always parents even if one doesn't get along with them. A story was told of a child visiting his grandparents. His grandmother had given him more sweets than his parents usually approved of, but it was noted that some parents feel that in a grandparent's house usual rules could occasionally be broken. It was suggested that grandparents like to do special things for their grandchildren, but realize the parents must make the daily decisions. It was stated that although disagreements are inevitable between parents and grandparents, adults could usually work things out.

Second, Donna's next visit home was planned in minute detail. Issues such as who would pick her up, would they call first, which staff member would be on, and what would staff do to prepare Donna for the visit were all negotiated. Problems that might arise were discussed. What if Donna became sick just before her parents were to pick her up? What if she became sick just before she was to be brought back to the residence? Participants were asked what could go wrong on the home visit that would interfere with Donna's treatment. Would the parents baby her?

The consultant at this point said that maybe they were moving too fast. The visit was to be an overnight. It was suggested that a 1-hour visit be planned instead, since overnights were unpredictable and could be disastrous. He stated that he was frightened and not really sure that these two groups of very concerned care-givers could really work together, since their views were so divergent. Donna may, he said, either have to live at home, requiring the parents to give up their retirement plans of traveling around the region selling antiques and requiring the staff to admit that they had failed with Donna, or have to live independently of her parents, requiring her to go to the workshop every day, return to the residence, watch TV, interact with staff socially, and give up her family ties. All parties assured the consultant that they could resolve any problems. It was again stated that moving more slowly and cautiously was indicated, but that they could try it if they all agreed. To accomplish this, the last part of the recommendation was that a biweekly meeting be convened by the case manager to iron out any difficulties that arose in the creation of this complementary decisional subsystem.

A final meeting was held with the case manager alone to process the intervention and to equip her with the family systems therapy techniques of positive connotation, prescription of the symptom, and restraint from change. At 3- and 6-month telephone follow-ups, the case manager reported that the arrangement was working well. A system of defined visits was established, as were guidelines for behaviors in each household. Donna continued her poor behavior, but no one escalated the responses. It was hoped that, eventually, the intervention would lead to a curtailment of the symptom; however, the consultant never suggested that the symptom would end. One year later, the symptoms had indeed disappeared. The meetings were taking place monthly, and the case manager had successfully used a similar approach in two other cases.

RECOMMENDATIONS

Decisional Subsystems

As family therapists work with cases of agency enmeshment, they obviously must expand their view of the boundaries of the unit of treatment.

Furthermore, just as family therapists sometimes choose to overtly ignore dynamics internal to individuals in families, it is sometimes important to ignore conflicts within families and within agencies in order to make an agency enmeshment dilemma manageable.

What has happened in this case that demonstrates a new role for the systemic family therapist? Certainly, the problem focus—a mentally retarded adult in a residential placement—is generally new for family therapists. The most important new function, however, is the construction of a decisional subsystem to ensure that the identified client's basic life decisions are made and carried out. A family therapy consultant's primary responsibility is to ensure that the members of the decisional subsystem, who represent all levels of all interactive systems (e.g., clients, their families, significant others, and service providers), have a complementary relationship. In answer to the question, of what system is this a subsystem, it is a subsystem of the larger context of social regulation and service systems interacting with their consumers and with each other.

A family therapist called in on a case focused on a mentally retarded adult within the larger service system can develop a decisional subsystem as part of the assessment process. Like any subsystem, its membership and functions may continue, change, or end over time. It is often helpful to meet separately with the major parties at first, as they see themselves as very separate systems. It is sometimes difficult for the consultant to determine who is meaningfully connected to the case and who can represent whom at the meetings. Circular questioning can be used to determine who is involved, to what extent, and at what point in the problem cycle. All departments and levels that affect treatment should be included in the decision making. It is not necessary and often not possible to remove any outside helpers from the case. If the consultant finds a way to identify clear complementary relationships between the parties, they will themselves eliminate the unneeded. The only outsider the consultant will want to remove is himself or herself.

A decisional subsystem is intended to make the involvement of the family therapy consultant as brief as possible. The operation of the subsystem with the consultant present is, therefore, limited to three basic functions: assessment, information giving, and decision making. First, it is useful for the consultant to conduct a thorough problem-focused interview with all the parties together to test out and elaborate on the hypotheses. Crucial to this aspect is finding ways that the parties' behavior can be framed as complementary. Bringing all the involved parties together can sometimes bring the problems out in the open, even if the consultant has carefully prepared the parties in the separate meetings. The consultant should be ready to recognize and manage any such problem.

Second, usually at a succeeding meeting, the consultant's view of the problem can be shared and additional information provided. A major task of any family therapist is to frame a situation in a manner that makes change possible. The systemic family therapy techniques of positive connotation, prescription of the symptom, and restraint from change are useful tools for the consultant who is beginning to build complementary relationships between the various parties.

Third, the parties need an opportunity to experience successful, cooperative decision making. The consultant must find a task that all can agree needs to be accomplished. It should be a minor or neutral task that does not appear to resolve any of the major conflicts, however, as initial change that is too significant or occurs too quickly can prohibit any progress at all. The consultant must not guide this third function of the subsystem.

The best person to be in charge of the meetings is often the professional helper most responsible for the overall coordination of the case. Frequently, this is the person who asked for help (although sometimes the family has asked for the help). This person usually has the power to convene everyone and the willingness to try something different to improve the situation. The question of how the hierarchy should be organized is not always so easily resolved, however.

It is important to clarify the hierarchical organization so as to define the roles of the subsystem members. Haley's (1980) and Madanes' (1981) views on hierarchy are well-known: parents should be in charge of children, therapists in charge of cases, and supervisors in charge of therapists. Simple power hierarchies, useful sometimes, are usually not practical in problems of agency enmeshment. In these cases, hierarchy must be more flexible and vary with the situation. At home, the parents must be in charge; at the residence, the staff must decide how to enforce the rules; and at subsystem meetings, the case manager must lead the decision-making process. Critical to the success of decisional subsystems is the use of a situational hierarchy.

Teaching Family Therapy

Another aspect of this new approach is its emphasis on teaching certain family therapy techniques and principles to case managers so they can guide the decisional subsystem on their own. Practical techniques such as positive connotation, prescription of the symptom, and restraint from change can be taught, first by example and later by direct discussion. To ensure that the techniques will be used safely, certain principles must also be taught. These include (1) how to identify the meaningful unit of treatment, (2) how to vary the hierarchy situationally, and (3) how to distinguish between the normative and unique developmental issues of these families.

Furthermore, the consultant helps the case manager understand that all parties are trying in their own way "to make the system work." The consultant remains available for questions, but must clearly transfer responsibility for the case back to the case manager.

CONCLUSION

In describing a new role for systemic family therapists, a case was presented to illustrate the unique therapeutic and developmental issues in families and larger systems organized around a mentally retarded adult. As retarded adults and others in custodial care become more frequently served by family therapists, the use of decisional subsystems can be an effective and efficient way to resolve conflicts and restore services to a useful role in development.

REFERENCES

Aponte, H.D. (1981). Structural family therapy. In A. Gurman & D. Kniskern (Eds.), *Handbook of family therapy*. New York: Brunner/Mazel.

Carter, E., & McGoldrick, M. (1980). *The family life cycle: A framework for family therapy*. New York: Gardner Press.

Coppersmith, E.I. (1983). The place of family therapy in the homeostasis of larger systems. In M. Aronson & R. Wolberg (Eds.), *Group and family therapy: An overview*. New York: Brunner/Mazel.

Goolishan, H., & Anderson, H. (1981). Including non-blood related persons in family therapy. In A. Gurman (Ed.), *Questions and answers in the practice of family therapy*. New York: Brunner/Mazel.

Haley, J. (1980). *Leaving home: The therapy of disturbed young people*. New York: McGraw-Hill.

Madanes, C. (1981). *Strategic family therapy*. San Francisco: Jossey-Bass.

Minuchin, S. (1974). *Families and family therapy*. Cambridge: Harvard University Press.

Selvini Palazzoli, M.S., Boscolo, L., Cecchin, G., & Prata, G. (1980). The problem of the referring person. *Journal of Marital and Family Therapy, 6*, 3–9.

Turner, A.L. (1980). Therapy with families of a mentally retarded child. *Journal of Marital and Family Therapy, 6*(2), 167–171.

Wolfensberger, W. (1972). *The principle of normalization in human services*. Toronto: National Institute on Mental Retardation.

12. A Special "Family" with Handicapped Members: One Family Therapist's Learnings from the L'Arche Community

Evan Imber Coppersmith

Acknowledgments: The author expresses her deep appreciation to the members of the L'Arche Community, Calgary, for their openness and cooperation with this research. Special thanks to Pat Lenon, Director, L'Arche Calgary, for facilitating this research effort in both words and actions, and to Lascelles Black for encouraging this project.

And yet community is what L'Arche is about. It is not an organization which believes in offering mentally handicapped people a form of care, however kindly. It is an organization which believes that we must go further than that, that we must try in whatever we can to break down the barriers of stereotyping and labelling. . . . It believes in sharing the details of everyday life with as much respect as we can muster for those who have been defined inadequate just as it believes in sharing work and leisure and joy and suffering. (Shearer, 1974, pp. 7–8)

As a systemic family therapist with an abiding interest in large human service systems and their impact on family and individual functioning, I am continually searching to discover those aspects of families and larger systems that facilitate rather than impede human development. On Christmas Day, 1982, I was invited to dinner at the L'Arche community, Calgary, Alberta. I found myself in a large room surrounded by approximately 50 adults of varying ages and a few children and teen-agers. Many of the adults had profound and visible handicaps, including mental retardation of varying degrees and physical handicaps that required wheelchairs and walkers. The general nature of the handicapped population was not new to me, but the tone of this gathering was different. The atmosphere was infused with mutual respect, caring, a great deal of humor, expressiveness, clear expectations of participation and responsibility, relatedness. Missing was the sense of despair, cynicism, burn-out, one-upmanship, or drudgery often seen in residential settings. Something was happening here that could not be attributed simply to Christmas. People were involved with one another in ways that I knew had implications for families with handicapped members and for human service delivery systems. I wanted to know more. What follows is a report, from a systemic perspective, of participant observation research with the L'Arche community, Calgary, conducted during 1983. Relevant connections to family therapy and larger system interaction with handicapped persons and their families will be highlighted.

L'ARCHE: A BRIEF HISTORICAL OVERVIEW

L'Arche, which means "the ark," began in 1964 in Northern France when its founder, Jean Vanier, opened his home to live communally with two men from a local psychiatric hospital. Today, L'Arche is an international federation with communities of handicapped adults and persons referred to as "assistants" in Europe, Canada, the United States, India, Africa, Australia, and Central America. Over 2,000 people are presently living with L'Arche, split nearly 50-50 between handicapped and assistants. The size of L'Arche communities varies from one house for 6 or 8 people to a community of 350 people living in 28 houses (*International Federation of L'Arche*, 1981).

Vanier began L'Arche out of a desire to create a community infused with Christian values, particularly the Beatitudes. This philosophy underpins L'Arche communities today. L'Arche quickly became ecumenical; the first community was primarily Catholic, the second Anglican, and the third Hindu. People of all religions are welcomed in L'Arche, and differences are both acknowledged and respected.

L'Arche communities differ widely, respecting the need to adapt to and interact with local customs, rather than require adherence to a rigid code that may not fit particular circumstances. A central goal of all L'Arche communities, however, is the creation and maintenance of relationships with people who are handicapped.

> L'Arche is special, in the sense that we are trying to live in a community with people who are mentally handicapped. Certainly we want to help them grow and reach the greatest independence possible. But before "doing for them," we want to "be with them"! (Vanier, 1979, p. IX)

It is this focus on the natural growth that can occur via *relationship* in all its aspects, including cognitive, affective, physical, and spiritual, that frequently obliterates distinctions between care-giver and care-receiver and sets L'Arche apart as a larger system with special interest for the family therapist.

L'ARCHE, CALGARY: A SYSTEMIC ANALYSIS

Every family or larger system with handicapped members is required to organize in ways that respond to the handicapping conditions. This becomes even more salient when the system's defined role is to work with handicapped persons. Beliefs about the handicapped, myths regarding capabilities, and specified roles abound in such systems and often become reified and attributed to the handicapped person, per se, rather than to particular contextual constraints. Here, L'Arche is unusual in that it recognizes its own contribution as a contextual force in the lives of its handicapped members and has struggled to create a context that facilitates growth and development without falling into the trap of demanding it.

L'Arche is a complex system, involving several levels of accountability, e.g., its government funding source, religious institutions, its own board of directors, and the families of those who live there. It is a system for the handicapped with multiple external connections that has not become mired in bureaucratic rigidities, but rather has maintained a developmental direction.

Boundaries

The boundaries between L'Arche and the outside world are carefully organized. New members, whether handicapped or assistants, are involved in a lengthy entry process that requires a commitment by the individual to the community and by the community to the individual for an agreed upon and renewable period of time. No one is simply "dumped" at L'Arche or forced to be there. People who would pose a physical danger to the existing community or themselves are not accepted into L'Arche. Nonetheless, people with fairly severe emotional and behavioral problems do enter L'Arche, with the community deciding what it is able to handle at a given point in time. While L'Arche notes information provided by prior settings, particular care is taken to avoid adopting labels and stigmatizing new people.

Boundaries between persons within the community are mediated by an explicit rule against secret alliances. Thus, if one member seeks a second member in order to talk about a third member, that second member is expected to send the person to speak directly with the third member. Gossip is avoided, and the confusion engendered by secret and denied coalitions is interdicted. Since handicapped adults have frequently been involved in intense triadic arrangements in their families of origin, this rule contravenes the easy repetition of familiar patterns. It is a seemingly simple rule, yet it is profound in its implications. Most handicapped adults have become accustomed to being talked about by others, rather than being talked to about issues that affect their lives. They may be accustomed to being secretly sided with by one parent against another parent or to being the intense focus of conflict between their family and outside professionals. Thus, it is a new and unexpected experience for them to be expected to work out their own relationships directly on a one-to-one basis. Responsibility for personal relationships and for one's contribution to the overall health of the system is a mark of mature and responsible adulthood not often expected of handicapped adults. Thus, the rule against secret alliances promotes both the welfare and the entire system and the individuals who comprise it.

The boundaries between L'Arche and those members who leave range from much continued involvement to a total severance, generally depending on the reasons for the departure and the desires of both the individual and the community. Many handicapped people leave L'Arche to assume more independent living. They may retain their membership in L'Arche and frequently participate in community events. Occasionally, the handicapped person opts for a greater distance, and this is respected.

If a person, either handicapped or assistant, consistently behaves in ways that seriously infringe on the rights of others and the community cannot manage this through ordinary or extraordinary consequences, that person is asked to leave. Unlike other organizations working with the handicapped, L'Arche does not assume responsibility for placing the person, such as by making a referral. Strong efforts are made to connect the person to family and other community resources, but L'Arche does not "follow" the person or make long-range recommendations to a new setting. Patterns of overinvolvement are thus avoided. L'Arche considers that those who go out on their own because of untenable behavior have made a decision to sever relationship with the community. While this practice may appear harsh at first, it actually functions to communicate respect and a belief that people are capable of making choices about their behavior. It also reduces enmeshment and invests energy in the existing community.

The impact of people entering or leaving the community, regardless of circumstances, is handled with great care. L'Arche is especially sensitive to the ways in which people leaving can affect handicapped persons, since they are likely to have experienced multiple losses in their lives. This impact is not ignored or denied. Even when the leaving is a relief at one level, aspects of guilt and grief are dealt with and respected. Disruptive, angry behavior is understood as a message about pain at the loss of a relationship. This is in sharp contrast to the often held myth about the mentally retarded, which equates low intellectual functioning with a lack of affective experience. L'Arche recognizes that retarded adults experience the domain of feelings deeply, even if it is difficult for them to express their feelings verbally.

L'Arche is open to input from nonmembers, as seen by its involvement with medical and psychiatric consultants, volunteers, board members, church personnel, family, and friends. However, such input is critically examined, rather than simply accepted. Experts are respected for their area of expertise, but the community retains a sense of knowing best about itself. Thus, an openness to new information is able to interact with a well-informed identity, allowing the community to develop in new ways, while remaining connected to core values.

L'Arche in Calgary maintains clear boundaries to the international L'Arche community through newsletters, cards to and from people who have moved to another community, and attendance at meetings with members of other communities. Members take trips and holidays at various geographical locations. This broadens the handicapped members' sense of connection to a larger community, indeed to other parts of the world. This is an unusual experience for most handicapped adults, who frequently live within narrow boundaries of family and geographical location, and again sets L'Arche apart as a system that recognizes a universal human need to experience a sense of connectedness to a larger and continuous context.

The rules regarding boundaries at L'Arche are not ideal for all systems with handicapped members. The specific boundary arrangements are probably less important than the fact that the spoken rules and the actual behavior are in harmony. Members know what they can rely on and are not mystified in the interactional sphere. Boundaries are organized to support both individual and community viability.

Symmetry and Complementarity

In families and larger systems with handicapped members, relationships are generally structured and viewed as complementary. The handicapped person is often frozen in such positions as follower, recipient of care, or perpetual learner while the so-called nonhandicapped person serves as leader, care-giver, or teacher. Opportunities for shifting this rigid complementarity or for achieving symmetry are often nonexistent, and the reified roles perpetuate one another. At L'Arche, definitions of complementarity and symmetry are more complex.

To begin, since all have made a commitment to a community that is larger than any one person, all are on the same level, or symmetrical, and in a complementary relationship to a greater good. This symmetry is embedded in common activities in which all participate, such as community meetings and prayer. During a weekly meeting in which all participate, everyone shares their schedule for the week, communicating that all are equally important, that all have appointments, etc. It is assumed at L'Arche that even the most handicapped individual can participate in a decision-making process. All committees are ad hoc, rather than standing, and handicapped members sit on committees with assistants. Both handicapped and assistants assume temporary leadership positions. Verbal expression of feelings is encouraged for all members. Since the emotional drain is shared by handicapped and nonhandicapped alike, this, too, contributes to a sense of symmetry in relationships.

While opportunities for symmetrical relationships exist and are valued, L'Arche does not operate with a phony sense of equality. Differences between the handicapped and the assistants are real, and complementary relationships abound. For instance, during a lengthy decision-making process on the structure of weekly meetings, handicapped persons were paired with assistants to discuss the issue. The assistants went to great lengths to be certain that the handicapped understood the issue and could vote on it. From the positions of teacher and learner, the issue was thrashed out, until a shift could be made so that all were engaged in the symmetrical act of voting.

There are times when the handicapped members assume positions of leadership, both formally, as in chairing committees, and informally. Assistants describe the blurring of the distinction between care-giver and care-receiver in their experience at L'Arche, frequently saying that they receive as much care as they give and that they are taught by the handicapped as much as they teach. Roles and hierarchy are flexible. In order to minimize rigid role definitions, a daily log book is not kept. The community is, hence, not divided into those who observe and write about others' behavior, and those whose behavior is observed and written about. In the same relationship, one can be parent, friend, teacher, or learner.

L'Arche has generated a flexible range of relationship definitions that makes both symmetrical and complementary relationships available to everyone in varying degrees and circumstances. The family therapist involved with families that have handicapped members often finds the system beset by complementary patterns that obviate growth and change. Interventions that facilitate greater symmetry and reverse rigid complementarity will likely allow development of all the system's members. Many of the L'Arche practices can be adapted to family functioning.

Use of Rituals

L'Arche makes extensive use of rituals to organize time and space, to define relationships among members and with God, and to highlight individual uniqueness. Daily rituals, such as prayer and the evening meal, and weekly rituals, such as community meetings and prayer evenings, define ongoing membership in the community, highlight connectedness and a sense of unity, illuminate that which is reliable and continuous in life, and provides an opportunity for celebration.

In a population that is often accustomed to negatives, rituals at L'Arche frequently underscore positives. In a population that others might consider had much to mourn, rituals at L'Arche often celebrate life. They are used to reframe life experiences in ways that focus on hope and joy, rather than on cynicism and despair. For instance, in the ritual called "Special Moments" each member describes one special moment of the preceding week. All listen, and all are oriented to notice the positive. Two rituals of particular importance are "Days of the Week" and the birthday celebration ritual.

"Days of the Week" is a scheduling ritual that takes place during the weekly meeting. Both the handicapped and the assistants announce their schedules for each day of the coming week. The ritual is led by one member who retains this job for a month. On one occasion when I witnessed this ritual, the leader had a severe speech difficulty and could barely say the days but she was supported and helped and expected to perform her part and she did. The process is lengthy, but full of humor. The effect of the ritual is complex. All are oriented to time and place together. Past, present, and future become viable concepts in a ritual of continuity. Everyone knows who is meeting with whom, eliminating concerns over secret alliances. The participation of everyone obliterates unnecessary hierarchical differences and affectations. In a world where adults who carry schedule books are seen as "important," everyone becomes an important person whose time is valuable.

The birthday ritual is used to celebrate each member's birthday in a way that highlights both individuality and connectedness to the larger community. The ritual begins with the birthday person telling the story of how he or she came to L'Arche. This story maintains a connection to a life prior to and outside of L'Arche, while at the same time underscoring the person's relationship to the community. Then, one at a time, the members tell the birthday person the way in which that person is a gift to them. Each statement starts "The gift you are to me" and concludes with a description of that person's qualities in relationship to self. Finally, the birthday person is asked to describe "the gift you are to yourself." For a handicapped person infused with negative beliefs about self, this aspect of the ritual is dramatic in that it requires new definitions of self. Only those people speak who wish to do so. I witnessed this ritual twice. Both times I observed the handicapped members expressing themselves in clearer speech and more complex thought and feelings than before or after the ritual. Intense emotions can be expressed within the safe boundaries of the ritual. Thus, permission is given both for silence and for the open expression of deep caring and affection.

Since ritual, per se, relies less on intellect and abstract verbalization, and more on metaphors and symbolic acts that can be used repetitively, providing room for improvisation is allowed, it is an excellent tool for families and larger systems with handicapped members, providing that improvisation is allowed. The ritual must grow out of the needs of the system, however, rather than being imposed on it. Thus, the L'Arche rituals work for L'Arche, but it is unlikely that they can simply be transposed to another setting. Rather, they are intended to stimulate the development of appropriate new rituals for families with handicapped members.

The Paradox of Acceptance and Change

Since "being with" is more important than "doing for" at L'Arche, it follows that accepting handicapped members as they presently are is more important than focusing on how they will be. L'Arche, thus, has no static, prearranged plans for development, time to leave, or independent living. As a larger system involved with handicapped members, L'Arche is unique and quite radical in this regard. Each individual is fully respected in his or her present state and not for some future, as yet unrealized, "potential." No one is "ordered" to grow or change at L'Arche. No one ever suggests, "In 6 months, you will do this, and in 12 months, you will do that." Yet, L'Arche members do change and grow, sometimes dramatically, sometimes beyond anyone's expectations. Many opt for independent living. Others choose to remain living in the community. Both choices are seen as equally valid.

For most handicapped adults, life has been a series of goals set by someone else, goals that communicate "you must be other than who you presently are" in order to be loved, accepted, or rewarded. The L'Arche community embodies the paradoxical elements described by systemic thinkers, for it is in the moment that the handicapped member is fully accepted as he or she is that genuine change and growth become possible. The L'Arche experience of being received, accepted, and respected as one is, paradoxically frees the person to grow and change.

IMPLICATIONS FOR THE FAMILY THERAPIST

During the time that this research was going on, the L'Arche community experienced both normative and idiosyncratic life cycle transitions. Two assistants married each other and left and the community celebrated their wedding. One handicapped member died in a tragic accident and the community mourned his death. One member was required to leave for behavior that was dangerous to the community. Other members moved to independent living. New handicapped members and new assistants were welcomed. Changes of this magnitude in so short a time period are stressful for any system. A system with handicapped members, for whom change can be quite threatening, can be severely stressed. As I witnessed L'Arche, Calgary, during this time period, however, the changes were recognized and accommodated. Stress was expected and accepted. Members were encouraged to talk about rather than act out their distress. A focus on positive development was maintained even during the most difficult times, while still allowing for the expression of pain and anger.

L'Arche has many practices that no doubt contribute to its capacity to live and work successfully with handicapped adults. While these various practices could be adopted by families and larger systems with handicapped members, L'Arche offers still more. It implicitly defines itself as an emergent system. Great care is taken when rules and patterns are changed. Processes are considered thoroughly and completed slowly enough so that the most handicapped member can participate with dignity. In this way, the change process is experienced and owned by all. For the family therapist working with families or larger systems with handicapped members, the clues to healthy development provided by L'Arche probably lie in its refusal to hammer out static goals, its battle to free itself from labels and stereotypes, its simultaneous embrace of both the present and the possible, and its view of itself as an evolutionary system.

REFERENCES

International Federation of L'Arche. (1981). Ontario: Daybreak.
Shearer, A. (1976). *L'Arche*. Ontario: Daybreak.
Vanier, J. (1979). *Community and growth: Our pilgrimage together*. Toronto: Griffin House.